Beyond the Bones

Academic Press is an imprint of Elsevier
125 London Wall, London EC2Y 5AS, UK
525 B Street, Suite 1800, San Diego, CA 92101-4495, USA
50 Hampshire Street, 5th Floor, Cambridge, MA 02139, USA
The Boulevard, Langford Lane, Kidlington, Oxford OX5 1GB, UK

British Library Cataloguing-in-Publication Data
A catalogue record for this book is available from the British Library

Library of Congress Cataloging-in-Publication Data
A catalog record for this book is available from the Library of Congress

ISBN: 978-0-12-804601-2

For Information on all Academic Press publications
visit our website at http://www.elsevier.com/

Working together
to grow libraries in
developing countries

www.elsevier.com • www.bookaid.org

Publisher: Sara Tenney
Acquisition Editor: Elizabeth Brown
Editorial Project Manager: Joslyn Chaiprasert-Paguio
Production Project Manager: Priya Kumaraguruparan
Designer: Maria Inês Cruz

Typeset by MPS Limited, Chennai, India

To my parents, who taught me to delight in the written word, and to Dr. Nancy Lovell, my first mentor in anthropology. Thank you all for your unwavering support and encouragement.

—Madeleine Mant

To my parents, who have supported me throughout this process and in all my other journeys.

—Alyson Holland

LIST OF CONTRIBUTORS

J. Bekvalac
Centre for Human Bioarchaeology, Museum of London, London, United Kingdom

C. de la Cova
Department of Anthropology, University of South Carolina, Columbia, SC, United States; African American Studies Program, University of South Carolina, Columbia, SC, United States

A. Holland
Department of Anthropology, McMaster University, Hamilton, ON, Canada

L. Lockau
Department of Anthropology, McMaster University, Hamilton, ON, Canada

M. Mant
Department of Anthropology, McMaster University, Hamilton, ON, Canada

S. Marciniak
Department of Anthropology, McMaster University, Hamilton, ON, Canada

A. Murphy
Faculty of Life Sciences, University of Manchester, Manchester, United Kingdom

K. Reusch
School of Archaeology, University of Oxford, Oxford, United Kingdom

M.A. Schillaci
Department of Anthropology, University of Toronto Scarborough, Toronto, ON, Canada

S. Wichmann
Leiden University Centre for Linguistics, Leiden University, Leiden, The Netherlands; Laboratory of Quantitative Linguistics, Kazan Federal University, Kazan, Russia

Beyond the Bones is a particularly apt title for this book, because this volume shows how we can reach beyond the remains of our ancestors into their actual lived experiences. This is increasingly achievable through accessing the range of methods available for scholars from a variety of disciplines and encompassing varied datasets. In tandem, this provides a platform for making this subject matter accessible to the interested public. As many of the chapters show, comparative analysis of different sets of data can be challenging, but this does not mean that it should not be attempted. The synthetic project, *Health and disease in Britain. From prehistory to the present day* (Roberts and Cox, 2003), indeed showed, albeit using only one dataset (skeletal reports), how it is necessary that skeletal report authors use the same analytical methods and present data similarly.

The subject matter of the chapters in this book is varied and provides "something for all." The extensive project of digital radiography at the Museum of London (Bekvalac) shows the "added value" of such work for enhancing knowledge and as a learning tool, not forgetting the challenges of the ethics of sharing such data widely. Lockau's focus on metabolic bone disease emphasizes the need to take heed of clinical understanding of these diseases and think about diagnosis on a scale of confident to cautious and, very importantly, the continued need to explore early stages of bone changes in the skeleton—rather than always referring to "classic" examples reflecting people who had experienced the disease for some time. A consideration of living people's perceptions of the quality and quantity of their food intake (Holland) reminds us that, when looking to the past, we can forget that our ancestors were individuals, as we are today, who had dietary beliefs and preferences specific to them but also their social context. Marciniak's approach to Roman health and well-being through ancient pathogen DNA analysis shows the benefits of such approaches that link historical, skeletal, and contextual data, especially the gaps in knowledge for any one of those datasets that may be filled by another. Historical data are also a focus for Mant, Murphy, and Reusch.

We learn what we do not know about trauma in an 18th/19th century London hospital through skeletal remains, and yet find that considering contemporary documents in tandem may tell us about the nuances of health care decision making (Mant). We find that infant mortality as seen in skeletons is not linked to climate, following correlation with many variables (Murphy), and are allowed to explore the world of castrated people in the past through Reusch's fascinating multidisciplinary study. Finally, and unusually for bioarchaeology, Schillaci and Wichmann consider linguistic and craniometric data to look at genetic relationships in a New Mexico Pueblo group, identifying that they did not "evolve" together.

While dealing with disparate datasets and subject matter, this welcome volume will provide bioarchaeologists with ideas and challenges for being holistic in their approach to understanding the past.

Dr. Charlotte Roberts
Department of Archaeology, Durham University,
Durham, United Kingdom
February 2016

ACKNOWLEDGMENTS

Our thanks to the many scholars who generously agreed to review the following papers and whose vibrant commentary and discussion made the review process a delight. Special thanks to Dr. Rachel Ives, who originally encouraged us to publish this work, and to Dr. Carlina de la Cova, who has been a champion of this project from its nascent stage. Thank you also to Dr. Ann Herring, Dr. Megan Brickley, and Dr. Andrew Nelson for the support and advice during this process.

CHAPTER *1*

Introduction

M. Mant and A. Holland
Department of Anthropology, McMaster University, Hamilton, ON, Canada

Anthropological investigations into questions concerning health, disease, and the life course in past and contemporary societies necessitate interdisciplinary collaboration. Tackling these "big picture" questions related to human health-states requires understanding and integrating social, historical, environmental, and biological contexts and uniting qualitative and quantitative data from divergent sources and technologies. The crucial interplay between new technologies and traditional approaches to anthropology necessitates innovative strategies that promote the emergence of new and alternate views.

While there is recognition within anthropology of the importance of a multifaceted approach to research design and data collection, more concrete examples of research questions, designs, and results that are produced through the integration of different methods are needed to provide guidance for future researchers and foster the creation of discourse for constructive critique. New and exciting narratives are being written in anthropology, but few volumes have yet been published that bring together these varied voices. In this volume we seek to explore how current research in physical anthropology is responding to the challenges posed by disparate datasets. The papers included in this book will illustrate and promote a discussion of the problems, limitations, and benefits of drawing upon and comparing datasets, while illuminating the many ways in which anthropologists are using multiple data sources to unravel larger conceptual questions in anthropology.

The papers in this volume were first presented as posters in the symposium *Beyond the Bones: Engaging with Disparate Datasets* in St Louis, Missouri at the 2015 meeting of the American Association of Physical Anthropologists. The authors, a selection of senior graduate

Beyond the Bones. DOI: http://dx.doi.org/10.1016/B978-0-12-804601-2.00001-6

students and established professionals, answered a call for papers concerning mixed methods approaches in physical anthropology. Their work highlights lines of evidence as varied as historical documents, digital radiography, ancient DNA, linguistic distance, and public health interviews.

Murphy and Mant's work illustrates the value of engaging with historical datasets. Murphy explores infant mortality in historic North America and the United Kingdom by examining cemetery reports. Mant highlights the differences in fracture frequencies between skeletal samples and contemporary hospital admission records to access aspects of human choice in seeking medical care in the past. Bekvalac highlights the applications of direct digital radiography and computed tomography scanning to the unique skeletal collections of the Museum of London, while Reusch integrates historical, medical, and paleopathological data to explore the history of castration. Marciniak describes the technique of direct shotgun sequencing in ancient DNA research to identify potential pathogens in paleopathological samples in tandem with historical documents. Schillaci and Wichmann provide an example of the possible integration of linguistic and bioarchaeological datasets. Lockau considers the contributions of clinical data to paleopathological studies of metabolic bone disease. Holland discusses the integration of qualitative and quantitative methods in studying the perceptions of young adults concerning their intake of calcium and vitamin D.

These varied voices wrestle with the inherent challenges involved in working with multiple lines of data, but each chapter demonstrates the benefits of allowing disparate datasets to speak in concert.

CHAPTER 2

Fifty Shades of Gray Literature: Deconstructing "High" Infant Mortality With New Data Sets in Historic Cemetery Populations

A. Murphy
Faculty of Life Sciences, University of Manchester, Manchester, United Kingdom

2.1 INTRODUCTION

Human mortality is a cornerstone in any study describing the lived experience of past populations. It is frequently assumed that mortality—particularly infant mortality—was much higher in ancient cultures than it is today (Caldwell, 1996; Caldwell and Caldwell, 2003; Chamberlain, 2006; Guy et al., 1997; Lewis and Gowland, 2007; Sainz de la Maza Kaufmann, 1997). Unfortunately, prior to the advent of organized record keeping, it is difficult to describe past mortality with confidence (Harding, 1998). Osteological samples from historic cemeteries are one underutilized source that are uniquely suited to analyze whether mortality derived from osteological evidence may be a reliable proxy of the true mortality for the population being studied for two reasons. Firstly, historic cemeteries often have associated burial records, against which osteological estimates of mortality can be compared (Swedlund and Herring, 2003). Secondly, the burial practices utilized are generally understood: namely to preserve the mortal remains of the community for eternity (Cherryson et al., 2012). Theoretically, this results in the creation of a representative population sample, which is also comparatively well preserved.

Although it might seem that the juxtaposition of historical records with excavated cemetery reports would be a well-trodden avenue of inquiry, few studies have attempted to engage with both (Grauer and McNamara, 1995; Lanphear, 1989; Saunders et al., 1995). Though both are very common types of record, they are unusual in that they are often overlooked and rarely perceived as complementary. Historic

Beyond the Bones. DOI: http://dx.doi.org/10.1016/B978-0-12-804601-2.00002-8

cemetery reports seem homogenous, but are diverse in their presentation, retention, and study (Boyle, 2015). Archival records may be lost
to memory, inaccessible, incomplete, or untranslated (Grenham, 2006;
Jolly, 2013; Wilkes, 2013). Both have much to offer one another.
Among other reasons, cemetery reports are an excellent source of
information on infant mortality and archival records contain a
bonanza of demographic information (Swedlund and Herring, 2003).
Together, they are filled with potential for answering numerous questions about past health and lifeways.

Infant mortality, or the proportion of infants who perish in the first
year of life per thousand born, is central to the study of any culture.
(Acsadi and Nemeskeri, 1970; Chamberlain, 2006; Lewis and
Gowland, 2007). It is one of the best predictors of the overall health of
any population (Meckel, 1990). In modern times, it ranges from as little as 0.02% in developed countries to as much as 50% in areas of the
developing world (Barbieri, 2001; Department of the Interior, 2012;
Kuehn, 2008; Matthews and MacDorman, 2007). Because the current
range of existing infant mortalities is quite wide, to say that past infant
mortality was "higher than at present" tells us very little without
further qualification.

This pattern of wide mortality ranges persists in the numerous studies prior to CE 1900 (Fogel, 1986, 2004; McKeown, 1976; Newman,
1906; Rüttimann and Loesch, 2012; Wrigley and Schofield, 1989).
These sources describe the effects of nutrition, hygiene, vaccination,
and urbanization on the mortality decline leading up to the modern
era. They also have recorded infant mortality percentages from the
teens to the mid-1920s in rural England with highs of ~40% in urban
areas (Lewis and Gowland, 2007; Newman, 1906; Wrigley and
Schofield, 1989). In contrast, estimates as low as 2–3% have been proposed for Colonial America, rising into the teens by the 1900s (Brosco,
1999; Mays, 2004). Variation has been perceived between countries
and between localities within a given country, yielding regional ranges
from below 10% to over 50% (Newman, 1906; Rüttimann and Loesch,
2012).

Prior to CE 1500, a lack of records causes mortality estimates to
become increasingly unreliable, leading archaeologists to look to alternate sources to approximate them. Medically primitive communities
are one possible proxy; for example, infant mortality from 12% to 21%

is recorded among the Amish and 20% among the !Kung (Acheson, 1994; Howell, 1979). Studies of ancient demography have also attempted to understand mortality in prehistoric or classical populations using ages derived either from burials or the incomplete textual sources that were available (Acsadi and Nemeskeri, 1970; Bagnall and Frier, 1994; Hassan, 1981; McKechnie, 1999; Russell, 1958; Scheidel, 2001). The ambiguous nature of ancient data coupled with misgivings about sampling have increasingly led researchers to recognize the value of comparing archaeological and textual sources (Lewis, 2002; Lewis and Gowland, 2007; Perry, 2007; Photos-Jones et al., 2008; Swedlund and Herring, 2003). Rare studies have compared mortality from individual historical cemetery samples to burial records (Grauer and McNamara, 1995; Lanphear, 1989; Saunders et al., 1995). These have found agreement between the two mortality estimates, suggesting that cemetery mortality may be an adequate proxy for burial records among juveniles. However, this is only descriptive of specific sites. In order to state more generally whether this is true, many more historic cemetery samples must be compared.

In a survey of infant mortality in excavated medieval cemeteries, Buckberry (2000) was able to demonstrate figures around 30%. While not as low as most modern infant mortality, this is not as high as the estimates of ~35−40% and above which have been postulated by archaeologists and historical demographers (Caldwell, 1996; Coale and Demeny, 1983; Hollingsworth, 1968; Lewis and Gowland, 2007). This study attempts a similar survey of excavated historical cemeteries which employ sufficiently narrow age-at-death categories to consider the differences between infant, child, and adult mortality from the UK and the US with the goal of determining: (1) the range of infant mortalities in excavated historic cemeteries; (2) how this range compares to known historic estimates of infant mortality; and (3) whether the appearance of infant mortality is strongly influenced by factors such as climatic region, urbanization, sample size, and population size/density.

2.2 MATERIALS AND METHODS

Seventy-three reports of excavated historic cemeteries from the US and the UK with sample sizes of ten or more were studied for their inclusion of relevant demographic data derived from osteological sources.

The use of small samples was unavoidable, given the scarcity of larger excavated cemeteries. To mitigate this, samples were aggregated in several ways to improve their representativeness. In addition to the availability of reports, sample size, and a minimum quality of osteological analysis sufficient to yield precise ages at death (see Buikstra and Ubelaker, 1994), two other factors guided sample selection. First, because of potential noise from racial and socioeconomic differences (ie, disruption to family groups during missionization, forced relocation, or slavery) only cemetery samples with large percentages of European ancestry were selected (Chamberlain, 2006). Second, only demographically inclusive samples were used (Chamberlain, 2006). This removes distortion caused by differential age-specific mortality patterns such as would be expected within cemeteries associated with age- and gender-selective establishments (eg, military institutions, poor houses, and hospitals).

The samples used in this study are enumerated in Tables 2.1−2.2. Seventy-three cemeteries had suitable sample size (≥ 10) and age categories to facilitate the comparison of infants (0−1.9 years), children (2−17.9 years), and adults (18+ years). Two cemeteries with no infants were studied for their child mortality and age-specific mortality. In addition to these general age groups, 19 North American cemeteries and all 23 British cemeteries utilized more precise (ie, age-specific) categories (0−1.9 years, 2−11.9 years, 12−17.9 years, 18−34.9 years, 35−49.9 years, and 50−99.9 years). Although infant mortality is usually defined as occurring in the first year of life only, and although 1-year intervals are typically used in the youngest cohorts for demographic purposes (Chamberlain, 2006), the variable age categories yielded from osteological recording in the cemetery reporting precluded this. In model populations where overall life expectancy is relatively low, the mortality in the youngest age group (0−1.9 years) should still be sufficiently high to enable their comparison with Model West life tables without distorting the effects of infant mortality (Coale and Demeny, 1983; United Nations, 1982). Such tables are experimentally derived mortality profiles for different population types in developing countries. Juxtaposition of osteological mortality against life tables indicates whether the mortality pattern of the sample falls into one of several realistic ranges, or whether it displays abnormal traits (Coale and Demeny, 1983).

Table 2.1 US Cemeteries Used in This Study, Cemeteries With Precise (Numeric) Age Categories Marked With an X

Cemetery	State	n =	Age-Specific	Cemetery	State	n =	Age-Specific
Big Neal Cove Cemetery	AL	68		Filhiol Mound	LA	16	
Becky Wright Cemetery	AR	10		Lane Memorial Hospital	LA	13	
Eddy Cemetery	AR	16		7 Rivers Cemetery	NM	45	X
Alameda Stone Cemetery	AZ	1166	X	Kearny Rd Cemetery	NM	21	X
LA Cemetery	CA	31		St Regis Cemetery	MO	42	
Woodville Cemetery	DE	10		Collings & Watkins Cemetery	OR	10	
Roughton Browne Cemetery	GA	14		Voegtly Cemetery	PA	555	X
Shockley Cemetery	GA	18		Shippenville Cemetery	PA	28	
Fuller Family Cemetery	GA	44		Blanchard Cemetery	RI	11	
Richmond County Cemetery	GA	11		State Institutional Ground	RI	60	X
Pine Ridge Cemetery	GA	14		Hampstead Cemetery	SC	344	X
Dubuque 3rd St	IA	811	X	Son Cemetery	SC	11	
Mitchell Rd Cemetery	IL	15		Mason Cemetery	TN	35	
Vandawerker Burials	IL	11		Read Family Cemetery	TN	27	
Old Irish Cemetery	IL	13		Ridley Cemetery	TN	47	X
Thurston Cemetery	IL	21		Dawson Cemetery	TX	63	X
Grafton Cemetery	IL	163	X	Tucker & Sinclair Cemetery	TX	12	
Bowling Cemetery	IL	199	X	Adam's Family Cemetery	TX	11	
Stellwagen Cemetery	IL	15		Coffey & Boothill Cemetery	TX	15	
Douthitt Cemetery	IN	11		Guinea Rd Cemetery	VA	34	X
Bennett Cemetery	KY	56	X	Wrenn-Hutchinson Cemetery	VA	43	X
Horse Park Cemetery	KY	31	X	Oliver Family Cemetery	VA	10	
Branham Cemetery	KY	24	X	Weir Family Cemetery	VA	24	
Campbell County Cemetery	KY	15		Evans Cemetery	WV	101	X
1st Cemetery of St Peter	LA	29	X	Reynold's Cemetery	WV	32	X

Table 2.2 UK Cemeteries Used in This Study					
Cemetery	Location	n =	Cemetery	Location	n =
King's Lynn Quakers	King's Lynn	32	St Peter	Wolverhampton	149
King's Lynn Baptists	King's Lynn	19	St Hilda	South Shields	183
St George	Bloomsbury	113	Chelsea Old Church	London	193
Kingston on Thames Quakers	Kingston on Thames	360	St Luke's Old St	London	891
St Peter Le Bailey	Oxford	172	Spitalfields	London	421
Baptist Chapel, Littlemore	Oxford	29	St Pancras	London	631
Poole Baptist Church	Poole	101	St Bride's, Fleet St	London	443
Sheffield Cathedral	Sheffield	165	New Churchyard, Broadgate	London	143
Carver St Methodists	Sheffield	130	St Benet Sherehog	London	187
St Paul's, Pinstone St	Sheffield	14	City Bunhill Burial Ground	London	239
St Martin in the Bullring	Birmingham	505	Crossbones Burial Ground	London	148
Priory Yard Baptists	Norwich	63			

Where intermediate age categories were used (eg, 10−13 years), or some individuals within the cemetery fell into a nominal class (ie, adult, infant, child), they were divided and apportioned into refined age categories. The number placed in each category using this method was weighted according to standard attritional mortality patterns; generally in historical populations this is a bimodal curve with the highest mortality peak in early infancy and a lesser peak at the point in middle adulthood where increased risk meets declining survivorship (Acsadi and Nemeskeri, 1970; Chamberlain, 2006). While this introduces the potential for slightly skewing the appearance of mortality within a discrete category to seem more demographically typical, it prevents the distortion of mortality across all categories by preserving the size of the sample and the ratios of broad age categories.

Many of the UK cemeteries had sample sizes of ≥100. Because the sample size from US cemeteries was often quite small, they were studied individually and then aggregated into 18 states for comparison with the overall UK trends. Studying both small and aggregated samples is useful as localized population trends can be masked in larger samples, such as censuses (Bagnall and Frier, 1994), yet archaeologists frequently need to understand the composition of the smaller cemeteries they work with. Thus, much can be learned if the mortality demonstrated in the small samples is in accord with that of the larger ones. United States cemeteries with sample sizes of 100 or more were also examined as a group, to ensure that conglomerating samples was not artificially creating the appearance of plausible, yet misleading mortalities. The aggregated states and their sample sizes are presented in Table 2.3. These states were then subdivided into five geographic regions: the Northeast; the Mid-Atlantic; the South; the Southwest; and the Midwest (Table 2.4).

Because of its comparatively small landmass, the UK was considered as a sixth single region. In addition to experimenting with an even larger sample size, this enabled the comparison of mortality by region, a strategy that may influence both attrition and skeletal preservation. Mortality may change by region owing to increased risk posed by epidemic, environmental factors, population density, and social factors

Table 2.3 Samples Aggregated by US State			
State	n =	State	n =
Alabama	68	Missouri	42
Arkansas	26	New Mexico	66
Arizona	1166	Pennsylvania	583
California	31	Rhode Island	71
Georgia	101	South Carolina	355
Illinois	437	Tennessee	123
Iowa	811	Texas	101
Kentucky	126	Virginia	111
Louisiana	58	West Virginia	128

Table 2.4 Samples Aggregated by Region				
Region	Climate	States	n =	Cemeteries n =
United Kingdom	Temperate Maritime	N/A	5280	23
Northeastern US	Humid Continental	DE, PA, RI	1321	5
Mid-Atlantic US	Humid Continental-Subtropical	KY, VA, WV	355	9
Southern US	Humid Subtropical	AL, AR, GA, LA, SC, TN	718	16
Midwestern US	Humid Continental	IL, IN, MO, IA	1301	10
Southwestern US	Humid Subtropical-Arid	AZ, NM, TX	1258	6

(Acsadi and Nemeskeri, 1970). Taphonomic preservation may alter with seasonal precipitation, soil drainage, and heating/freezing cycles (Buckberry, 2000).

2.3 RESULTS

2.3.1 General Infant Mortality

Infant mortality in the UK cemeteries ranged from 2% to 50% (Fig. 2.1). In the 18 aggregated US states, it ranged from 3% to 46% (Fig. 2.2). More than two-thirds of the UK groups had an infant mortality (0–1.9 years) of 13% or below (Fig. 2.3). The remainder were ~20% and above, with a small group of outliers between 35% and 50%. Child mortality ranged from 6% to 28% with dual modes of 16% and 20%. Though averages for both infant and child mortality were 16%, the majority of samples displayed child mortality of ≥15% and infant mortality of ≤15%.

By contrast, average aggregated US infant mortality was 25%. This closely matched the profile of the nonaggregated cemeteries, showing that sample size was not the prime determinant guiding the appearance of mortality. Three discrete ranges of mortality clusters make a broad distribution from 10% to 25%, a peak at ~30–35% and a few higher

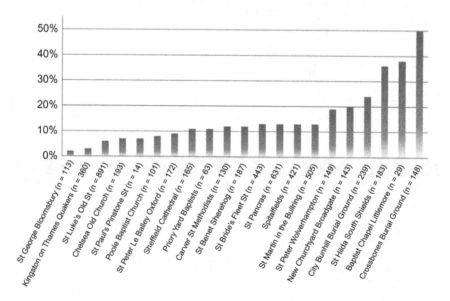

Figure 2.1 Infant (0–1.9 years) mortality in 21 UK cemeteries.

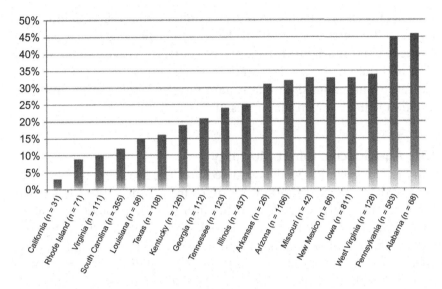

Figure 2.2 Infant (0–1.9 years) mortality in 18 aggregated US States.

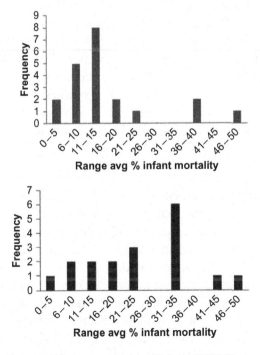

Figure 2.3 Histogram of frequency of average percent infant mortality in the UK (Top) and the US (Bottom).

outliers (Fig. 2.3). This pattern was visible in both the individual and aggregated comparisons. Within the 47 US cemeteries which included children, child mortality ranged from 3% to 53%, with an average of 25%, and dual modes of 19% and 29%. The range of child mortalities was more continuous than infant mortality, with the only slight differentiation being between the ranges of 10−25%, and 30−40%.

2.3.2 Age-Specific Infant Mortality

Forty-two cemeteries were examined for age-specific mortality and compared to expected mortality profiles from Model West life tables. A typical attritional mortality profile in a historic population displays a bimodal curve with the greatest peak during infancy (0−1.9 years), and a smaller peak at the most typical age of death in adulthood (anywhere between 35 and 80 years). Common variations in such profiles include a peak in early childhood (~2−5 years) in tandem with, or in lieu of a peak in infancy. Either infant or early childhood peaks may also be accompanied by a peak in early adulthood (18−30 years).

In comparison with life tables, all but four cemeteries could be fitted to a model with some accuracy. The most common were Levels One, Five, and Nine, with average life expectancy at birth (E0) between 20 and 40 years and annual growth rate (r) of 0.5%. All plausible mortality cemeteries exhibited either peaked infant mortality, peaked child mortality, or a combination of peaked infant/child mortality and peaked early adult mortality. Irregular mortality profiles were linear (ascending). Three examples of the commonly occurring plausible mortality profiles, and an example of an unlikely linear profile, are shown in comparison with a Level Five Model West profile in Fig. 2.4.

A summary of the modality of the different mortality curves for US and UK cemeteries is presented in Table 2.5. Fewer UK cemeteries had strong peaks in infant mortality than in the US. Of the US cemeteries with infant mortality peaks, 37% had corresponding peaks in early adult (18−34.9 years) mortality. In contrast, the UK had more cemeteries exhibiting heightened child mortality (52%), of which 30% also displayed peaks in early adulthood. Only 16% of US cemeteries had high peaks in child mortality, and 5% had corresponding peaks in early adult mortality. The overall percentage of early adult mortality was 10% higher in the US than the UK. The remainder of the cemeteries displayed variable geriatric mortality at 35 years or above.

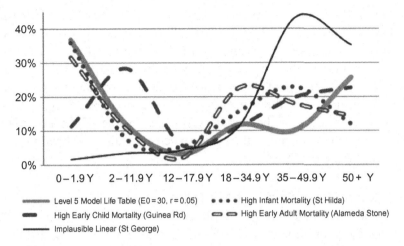

Figure 2.4 Examples of three plausible mortality profiles and one abnormal profile derived from cemeteries studied.

Table 2.5 Percent of the Population Expressing Age-Specific Modality (Peak) Combinations in Cemetery Mortality Profiles							
	Infant/ Geriatric (%)	Child/ Geriatric (%)	Infant/ Early Adult (%)	Child/ Early Adult (%)	Infant and Child/Early Adult (%)	Slightly Linear (%)	Strongly Linear (%)
US	37	16	37	5	–	–	5
UK	22	22	4	17	13	9	13

Few cemeteries in either country had abnormally strong ascending linear mortality profiles arising from a veritable exclusion of infants and lesser inclusion of children, along with an incremental increase in the adult age categories. These profiles are suggestive of an underenumeration of the young owing to age-specific burial exclusion or taphonomic loss. The remainder of profiles show mortality peaks in the following periods: (1) death in early infancy (prior to a year); (2) death in late infancy/early childhood (around 2–3 years); (3) most common age(s) of death in adulthood.

In those cemetery reports where more precise aging was used, and comparison with burial records was possible, infant death often occurred before the sixth month. Early child death commonly occurred late in the first year to the middle of the second year. Congenital factors or unsanitary birthing practices are often implicated in deaths within the first 6 months (Acsadi and Nemeskeri, 1970; Kuehn, 2008;

Meckel, 1990; Newman, 1906), and may be primarily responsible for the first of these mortality categories. Between the ages of 6 months and 4 years, unsanitary weaning practices are a common cause of death (Newman, 1906); the second mortality category likely includes many of these. Accident, respiratory ailment, or epidemic is increasingly implicated after the age of 3 or 4 years; however, fewer of these deaths were evident in the cemetery samples. Some of the urbanizing and frontier environments did exhibit such mortality profiles, perhaps suggesting these causes.

2.3.3 Region-Specific Infant Mortality
To explore the possibility that taphonomic factors may strongly influence cemetery preservation (Buckberry, 2000; Djuric et al., 2011), or that mortality patterns may correlate with climatic conditions which alter the spread of epidemics (Acsadi and Nemeskeri, 1970; Newman, 1906), infant mortality was studied by region. The US was divided into five geoclimatic regions, and compared to the UK as a whole. Average infant and child mortality by region is presented in Fig. 2.5.

The range of infant mortalities (0–1.9 years) was similar in all areas apart from the Southwest US, which began at a higher percentage and was around half the range of every other region. Maximum infant mortality was similar in all areas. The range of child mortalities

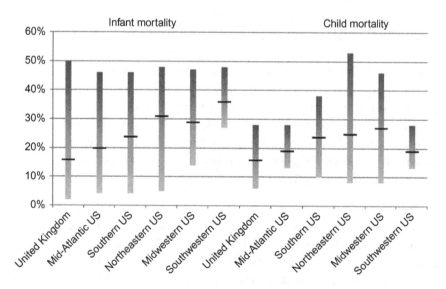

Figure 2.5 Range of infant and child mortality and their averages by region.

(2–17.9 years) was consistent in its minimum across all regions, but varied over 20% at its maximum between regions. Typically, the range of child mortality was narrower than the corresponding region's infant mortality. Both average infant and child mortality were lowest in the United Kingdom, however its range was greatest and highest in this area.

Average infant mortality was highest in the Southwest United States. Average infant and child mortality were similar to one another within the UK, the Midwest, and the Southern US. In other regions, infant mortality differed from child mortality. No two regions shared the same average infant mortality.

There was no obvious correlation between region and the appearance of infant or child mortality. For infant mortality, the coldest regions (UK and the Northeast) had similar ranges, but drastically different averages. This range was also similar to the much hotter Southern US, and the transitional Mid-Atlantic. The hottest regions (Southern and Southwest US) had dissimilar ranges and averages.

2.4 DISCUSSION

Average infant mortality for the US was 25% and 16% for the UK. The range of infant mortalities observed was almost identical between the UK (2–50%) and the aggregated samples from the US (3–46%). Figures on the lower end of this spectrum are somewhat unlikely given what is known about birth rates and living conditions in pre-Jennerian populations, that is, those prior to the widespread use of inoculation (Barbieri, 2001; Monnier, 2001). Despite this, the most commonly occurring infant mortalities ($\sim$10–35%) are on average lower than the "high" estimates previously believed. The outlying high mortalities (above $\sim$35%) are still realistic, but may represent more catastrophic circumstances (Acsadi and Nemeskeri, 1970; Meckel, 1990; Newman, 1906). It is likely that some loss occurs to cemeteries through taphonomy and partial sampling, meaning that even plausible observed mortalities are not a perfect representation of the buried group (Buckberry, 2000; Murphy, forthcoming). Furthermore, this shows that a variety of possible mortalities may be witnessed at different sites.

Typically a 10–15% difference between at least two distinct ranges of infant mortalities was seen in intercemetery comparisons.

Sixty-seven percent of the UK samples had an infant mortality of $\geq 10\%$, with 48% of all samples falling between 10% and 20% infant mortality. A second cluster of three samples had comparatively high mortalities (35–50%). The remaining 30% of samples fell just under 10%, suggesting underenumerated infants. The US was split more clearly into two distinct ranges, with a small quantity of samples in a third, high mortality group. Thirty-nine percent of aggregated US samples had an infant mortality of 30–35%, while 33% demonstrated an infant mortality of 10–20%.

These wide ranges and apparent mortality clusters suggest that separate mortality profiles exist within different geographically proximal groups and perhaps within individual population types. The specific cause of these varying profiles is not clear. One possibility is cemetery composition. In a small family cemetery, one might expect to find a disproportionate number of the very young and the very old as those of reproductive age migrate away, and perhaps migrate back for burial in their later years (Chamberlain, 2006). In a newly expanding city, an increased number of the unmarried may skew the composition of the population to early adulthood. Different environments may affect mortality in unpredictable ways: in urban settings, crowding and pollution may be combatted to some extent by access to work and modern amenities, whereas in frontier towns, lack of infrastructure, lawlessness, and lack of medical attention may negate the benefits of living space (Meckel, 1990; Newman, 1906). Additionally, within any community, the economic status of those buried may affect their mortality either through deficiency diseases, professional hazards, epidemics, or diseases of excess (Acsadi and Nemeskeri, 1970).

These statements are borne out to some extent by the examination of more detailed age-specific mortality profiles within cemeteries. Closer examination yielded peaks in mortality at different ages, which could often be understood in terms of lifestyle factors described in the associated reports. These include the presence of certain epidemics, pressures from urbanization, cemetery use-duration, and interpersonal violence. A variety of disparate yet plausible age-specific mortalities were thus observed in samples of different sizes. The mortality shifts most commonly witnessed were threefold. First, mortality was observed to vary in early childhood between neonatal, later infant, and early childhood mortality. This is likely owing to congenital disease and birthing practices in the first group, weaning hazards in the second, and risk of accident and epidemic in the third case (see Acsadi and Nemeskeri, 1970; Meckel, 1990; Rüttimann and Loesch, 2012). Secondly, in many samples, mortality rose prematurely in early adulthood. This may correspond with violence, dangerous professions, or parturition risks to women (Acsadi and Nemeskeri, 1970; Heilen and Gray, 2010). Finally, the average age of the geriatric differed somewhat across all samples.

Of the 19 US cemeteries with age-specific mortalities, only three (5%) had moderately "abnormal" mortality profiles. These cemeteries display almost linear increases in mortality, typical of age-preferential burial inclusion. The fact that they are geographically distant from one another, with other "regular mortality" cemeteries closer by, argues against purely taphonomic explanations. Twenty-two percent of UK samples demonstrated atypical mortality profiles, however only two of these (9%) were strongly linear. This pattern also correlates with Baptist and Quaker burial practices rather than with preservation influences. In the UK, average early childhood mortality was slightly higher than in infancy. Across the US, death in infancy was more common. In both countries, there appears to be a minor correlation between infant/child death and death in early adulthood, perhaps suggesting a link between loss of caregiver or contagion as a cause of early life mortality.

There was a minor positive correlation between sample size and higher infant mortality in the US. Most US cemeteries with an individual sample size of ≥ 100, as well as aggregated states, had an infant mortality of 30% or greater. However this trend was not linear; the largest cemeteries did not demonstrate the highest mortalities, nor did all large cemeteries display high mortality. Despite larger UK sample sizes, no corresponding correlation was observed. Though infant mortality ranged from 2% to 50%, four of the largest samples shared an infant mortality of only 13%. This suggests that factors like population growth and social-environmental conditions may correlate with heightened infant mortality, rather than increased mortality being an artifact of sample size. For example, although derived from a more populous city than remote Santa Fe or industrializing Pittsburgh, London samples in this study often demonstrated lower mortality.

No strong link could be found between climatic region and infant mortality. As previously noted, a wide range of infant and child mortalities was observed across both countries. This was also true across geographic areas. The wider range and generally lower averages of infant mortalities in long-settled areas, compared to the frontiers of the Midwest and the Southwest may suggest that perhaps settlement patterns are a greater indicator of mortality risk than climate itself. The western communities were rapidly expanding cities on the out-skirts of "civilization," while more easterly regions may have had greater infrastructure. Likewise, the higher early life mortality in the US as compared to the UK may have arisen from the more recent industrialization and changing migration patterns of the US.

2.5 CONCLUSIONS

In the past, it has been common to assume that infant mortality observed in an isolated excavated cemetery is either higher or lower than the "true" mortality of the buried population. The comparison of these similar, yet "disparate" datasets has clarified the complexity behind populations displaying identical mortalities with different causes, and identical environments that display opposite mortalities. Average infant and child mortalities in historic cemetery samples are 25% in the US and 16% in the UK. A variety of realistic mortality profiles exist within the large range of these groups, with characteristic variations occurring between infant, child, and early adult mortality peaks. Infant mortality figures of <10% are less likely. However figures of around 10–35% may be typical of the period; this corresponds with the findings of historical demographers (Newman, 1906; Rüttimann and Loesch, 2012; Wrigley and Schofield, 1989). No apparent correlation exists between climatic region and the appearance of infant mortality. Together, these factors imply that taphonomic factors may not have the strong negative effect on infant preservation once thought, and that climatic factors are not the primary determinant of infant mortality. There is a minor association between larger urban samples and infant mortality. Coupled with the heightened mortality in newer, expanding communities, this may suggest that settlement patterns, man-made environmental factors, and population growth are the biggest predictors of infant mortality.

In an attempt to reduce the variables present in this study, only cemeteries with high percentages of European ancestry, and so-called "normal" populations were included. It would be worthwhile to extend this study to see whether the appearance of mortality differs dramatically in other types of populations. While numerous factors may influence the appearance of mortality within a cemetery, most are dependent on too many variables to confidently state causality in this study (Chamberlain, 2006). The most prominent of these are probably prior cemetery disturbance and differential skeletal preservation, which both have the potential to impact the question, yet are difficult to quantify (Buckberry, 2000; Djuric et al., 2011; Lewis and Gowland, 2007). It was beyond the purview of this project to thoroughly assess the different environmental and socioeconomic circumstances of each cemetery group. It would be useful to compare these cemeteries to censuses and historical records for a more thorough understanding of the dynamics that may be responsible for different mortality profiles. Finally, taphonomic factors play an important role in the preservation of cemetery samples and the data that can be gleaned from them (Buckberry, 2000; Djuric et al., 2011; Lewis and Gowland, 2007). More in-depth study of the effect that preservation has upon the appearance of mortality is necessary to be confident that cemetery mortalities are reliable.

This study clearly shows that historic cemetery reports and archival records are rich sources of data for addressing questions about past cultures. With a relatively small sample, it was possible to explore mortality by age, region, climate, sample size, and social structure. These are only a few areas of inquiry that can be addressed with these "disparate datasets." Historically, such sources have been overlooked, or have not been combined. This is because researchers are constrained by the perception that only certain datasets fall within their specialization, or they become preoccupied with cultivating new methods and projects in search of "new data." Datasets need not be novel or radical to be profoundly useful; often reopening "long-resolved" debates using a fresh perspective and overlooked sources is sufficient.

REFERENCES

Acheson, L.S., 1994. Perinatal, infant, and child death rates among the Old Order Amish. Am. J. Epidemiol. 139, 173–183.

Acsadi, G.Y., Nemeskeri, J., 1970. History of the Human Lifespan and Mortality. Akademiai Kiado, Budapest.

Bagnall, R.S., Frier, B., 1994. The Demography of Roman Egypt. Cambridge University Press, Cambridge.

Barbieri, M., 2001. Infant and child mortality in the less developed world. In: Smelser, N.J., Baltes, P.B. (Eds.), International Encyclopedia of the Social and Behavioral Sciences. Pergamon, Oxford, pp. 7404–7410.

Boyle, A., 2015. Approaches to post-medieval burial in England: past and present. In: Tarlow, S. (Ed.), The Archaeology of Death in Post-Medieval Europe. Walter de Gruyter GmbH & Co., Berlin, pp. 39–60.

Brosco, J.P., 1999. The early history of the infant mortality rate in America: 'a reflection upon the past and a prophecy of the future'. Pediatrics 103, 478–485.

Buckberry, J., 2000. Missing, Presumed Buried? Bone Diagenesis and the Underrepresentation of Anglo Saxon Children. Assemblage: University of Sheffield Graduate School Journal of Archaeology, 5. Accessible: <http://www.assemblage.group.shef.ac.uk/5/buckberr.html>.

Buikstra, J.E., Ubelaker, D.H. (Eds.), 1994. Standards for Data Collection from Human Skeletal Remains. Arkansas Archaeological Survey Research Series No. 44. University of Arkansas Press, Arkansas.

Caldwell, J.C., Caldwell, B.K., 2003. Pretransitional population control and equilibrium. Pop. Stud.-J. Demog. 57, 199–215.

Caldwell, P., 1996. Child survival: physical vulnerability and resilience in adversity in the European past and the contemporary Third World. Soc. Sci. Med. 43, 609–619.

Chamberlain, A., 2006. Demography in Archaeology. Cambridge University Press, Cambridge.

Cherryson, A., Crossland, Z., Tarlow, S., 2012. A Fine and Private Place: The Archaeology of Death and Burial in Post-Medieval Britain and Ireland, vol. 22. University of Leicester Archaeology Monograph, Leicester.

Coale, A.J., Demeny, P., 1983. Regional Model Life Tables and Stable Populations. Academic Press, London.

Department of the Interior, United States Bureau of the Census, 2012. Historical Statistics of the United States, Colonial Times to 1957: Continuation to 1962 and Revisions. U.S. Dept. of Commerce, Bureau of the Census, Washington, D.C., 1965.

Djuric, M., Djukic, K., Milovanovic, P., Janovic, A., Milenkovic, P., 2011. Representing children in excavated cemeteries: the intrinsic preservation factors. Antiquity 85, 250–262.

Fogel, R.W., 1986. The nutrition and decline in mortality since 1700: preliminary findings. In: Engerman, S.L., Gallman, R.E. (Eds.), Long-Term Factors in American Economic Growth. Cambridge University Press, Cambridge, pp. 439–556.

Fogel, R.W., 2004. The Escape from Hunger and Premature Death: Europe, America, and the Third World. Cambridge University Press, Cambridge.

Grauer, A.L., McNamara, E.M., 1995. A piece of Chicago's past: exploring childhood mortality in the dunning poorhouse cemetery. In: Grauer, A.L. (Ed.), Bodies of Evidence: Reconstructing History Through Skeletal Analysis. Wiley-Liss, New York, pp. 91–103.

Grenham, J., 2006. Tracing Your Irish Ancestors. Genealogical Publishing Company, Dublin.

Guy, H., Masset, C., Baud, C.A., 1997. Infant Taphonomy. Int. J. Osteoarchaeol. 7 (3), 221–229.

Harding, V., 1998. Research priorities: an historian's perspective. In: Cox, M. (Ed.), Grave Concerns: Death & Burial in England 1700-1850. Council for British Archaeology, London, pp. 205–212.

Hassan, F.A., 1981. Demographic Archaeology. Academic Press, London.

Heilen, M., Gray, M., 2010. Deathways and Lifeways in the American Southwest: Tucson's Historic Alameda-Stone Cemetery and the Transformation of a Remote Outpost into an Urban City. Volume II: History, Archaeology, and Skeletal Biology of the Alameda-Stone Cemetery. Statistical Research Inc., Tucson.

Hollingsworth, T.H., 1968. The importance of the quality of the data in historical demography. Daedalus 97, 415–432.

Howell, N., 1979. Demography of the Dobe !Kung. Aldine de Gruyter, New York.

Jolly, E., 2013. Tracing Your Ancestors Using the Census: A Guide for Family Historians. Pen & Sword Books Ltd., Barnsley.

Kuehn, B.M., 2008. Infant mortality. JAMA-J. Am. Med. Assoc. 300, 2359.

Lanphear, K.M., 1989. Testing the value of skeletal samples in demographic research: a comparison with vital registration samples. Int. J. Anthropol. 4, 185–193.

Lewis, M.E., 2002. Impact of industrialization: comparative study of child health in four sites from medieval and postmedieval England (A.D. 850–1859). Am. J. Phys. Anthropol. 119, 211–223.

Lewis, M.E., Gowland, R., 2007. Brief and precarious lives: infant mortality in contrasting sites from medieval and post-medieval England (AD 850–1859). Am. J. Phys. Anthropol. 134, 117–129.

Matthews, T.J., MacDorman, M., 2007. Infant Mortality Statistics from the 2004 Period Linked Birth/Infant Death Data Set. National Vital Statistics Reports. U.S. Department of Health and Human Services, Center for Disease Control and Prevention, National Center for Health Statistics, Atlanta.

Mays, D.A., 2004. Women in Early America: Struggle, Survival, and Freedom in a New World. ABC-CLIO, New York.

McKechnie, P., 1999. Christian grave-inscriptions from the Familia Caesaris. J. Ecclesiast. Hist. 50, 427–441.

McKeown, T., 1976. The Modern Rise of Population. Academic Press, New York.

Meckel, R.A., 1990. Save the Babies: American Public Health Reform and the Prevention of Infant Mortality 1850-1929. Johns Hopkins University Press, Baltimore.

Monnier, A., 2001. Infant and child mortality in industrialized countries. In: Smelser, N.J., Baltes, P.B. (Eds.), International Encyclopedia of the Social and Behavioral Sciences. Pergamon, London, pp. 7398–7404.

Murphy, A., Forthcoming. Publishing the Perished: Uniform Collection Standards and the Future of Historic Cemetery Excavations in the United States. Unpublished Doctoral Thesis. University of Manchester Faculty of Life Sciences.

Newman, G., 1906. Infant Mortality: A Social Problem. The New Library of Medicine, London.

Perry, M.A., 2007. Is bioarchaeology a handmaiden to history? Developing a historical bioarchaeology. J. Anthropol. Archaeol. 26, 486–515.

Photos-Jones, E., Dalglish, C., Coulter, S., Hall, A., Ruiz-Nieto, R., Wilson, L., 2008. Between archives and the site: the 19th-century iron and steel industry in the Monklands, Central Scotland. Post-Mediev. Archaeol. 42, 157–180.

Russell, J.C., 1958. Late Ancient and Medieval Population. Transactions of the American Philosophical Society. New Series. The American Philosophical Society, Philadelphia.

Rüttimann, D., Loesch, S., 2012. Mortality and morbidity in the city of Bern, Switzerland, 1805–1815 with special emphasis on infant, child and maternal deaths. Homo 63, 50–66.

Sainz de la Maza Kaufmann, M., 1997. Contraception in three Chibcha communities and the concept of natural fertility. Curr. Anthropol. 38, 681–687.

Saunders, S.R., Herring, D.A., Boyce, G., 1995. Can skeletal samples accurately represent the living populations they come from? The St. Thomas' cemetery site, Belleville, Ontario. In: Grauer, A.L. (Ed.), Bodies of Evidence: Reconstructing History Through Skeletal Analysis. Wiley-Liss, New York, pp. 69–89.

Scheidel, W., 2001. Progress and problems in Roman demography. In: Scheidel, W. (Ed.), Debating Roman Demography. Brill, Leiden, pp. 1–83.

Swedlund, A.C., Herring, A., 2003. Human biologists in the archives: demography, health, nutrition, and genetics in historical populations. In: Herring, D.A., Swedlund, A.C. (Eds.), Human Biologists in the Archives. Cambridge University Press, Cambridge, pp. 1–10.

United Nations, 1982. Model Life Tables for Developing Countries. Department of International Economic and Social Affairs. United Nations Publications, Washington D.C., Population Studies No. 77.

Wilkes, S., 2013. Tracing Your Ancestors' Childhood: A Guide for Family Historians. Pen & Sword Press, Ltd., Barnsley.

Wrigley, E.A., Schofield, R.S., 1989. The Population History of England 1541–1871. Cambridge University Press, Cambridge.

CHAPTER 3

Direct Digital Radiographic Imaging of Archaeological Skeletal Assemblages: An Advantageous Technique and the Use of the Images as a Research Resource

J. Bekvalac
Centre for Human Bioarchaeology, Museum of London, London, United Kingdom

3.1 INTRODUCTION

The Museum of London, London, United Kingdom (MoL) is faced with the complicated task of maintaining archives of large and diverse skeletal collections. The collections have been recorded over the years in a variety of ways and the resultant data stored in a range of formats, from traditional paper records to early incarnations of electronic recording systems. The Centre for Human Bioarchaeology (CHB) at the MoL curates extensive collections of archaeologically-derived human skeletal remains from the Prehistoric, Roman, Anglo-Saxon, Medieval, and Post-Medieval time periods. The skeletal collections curated at the CHB are captured in a broad range of integrated digital methods, including databases, photographs, radiographs, and computed tomography (CT) scans. These methods have extremely advantageous applications, but there are also concerns with the implications of long-term sustainability in a world of rapidly changing technologies. The importance of using multiple modalities to record these collections is that they are each designed to capture a different type of data, which then presents the option of examining a single, large collection using multiple lines of evidence. Studies that might have previously focused only on a single methodology can now incorporate data that speak to multiple aspects of the same question, creating more efficient and holistic explorations of these unique skeletal collections.

Beyond the Bones. DOI: http://dx.doi.org/10.1016/B978-0-12-804601-2.00003-X

3.2 OSTEOLOGICAL DATABASE

The initial digitization of the MoL skeletal collections was the result of the large-scale excavations (1998–2001) at Spitalfields Market (Thomas, 2004). Excavations of the market uncovered the monastic site of St Mary Spital and revealed over 14,000 medieval skeletal remains, of which 10,500 are curated at the MoL (Connell et al., 2012; Thomas, 2004). The prospect of analysis of such an unparalleled number of skeletal remains precipitated the development of a new electronic database system (Fig. 3.1); the skeletal remains were also to be retained as part of the archaeological archive. Osteologist Brian Connell and IT specialist Dr. Peter Rauxloh devised and created a bespoke osteological database for recording and retaining the large osteological dataset, leading to the creation of a rapid recording system (Connell and Rauxloh, 2003), an osteological method statement (Powers, 2012), and the Wellcome Osteological Research Database (WORD) supported on an Oracle platform. The Oracle platform allows for the maintenance of large datasets, enabling the creation of a dynamic search engine and a powerful tool for recording, research, and conservation.

Funding in 2003 awarded by the Wellcome Trust established the CHB and funded a team of osteologists to analyze skeletal remains from earlier excavated sites in the City of London and Greater London Area. Between 2003 and 2007 there were two osteological teams, the developer-funded Spital team and the Wellcome-funded team, working in tandem to record the osteological data into the WORD using the same methods and standards for osteological recording (Brickley and McKinley, 2004; Buikstra and Ubelaker, 1994). The launch of the CHB website in 2007 marked the sharing of osteological data at a scale no other institution curating skeletal remains had previously achieved. It also allowed for the production of a groundbreaking publication in bioarchaeology (Connell et al., 2012), based upon the data of over 5000 individuals recorded and analyzed from St Mary Spital.

The CHB curates the skeletal remains of c.20,000 individuals and the WORD holds records for over 16,000 individuals. The digitized osteological data are freely shared, allowing researchers worldwide to create direct comparative studies. In addition to those accessing the datasets remotely, annually over 50 researchers visit the CHB to collect data. There has been a profound impact on the field of osteology; in fact, this ready access has caused a noticeable London bias in the osteological output of studies (Roberts and Mays, 2011).

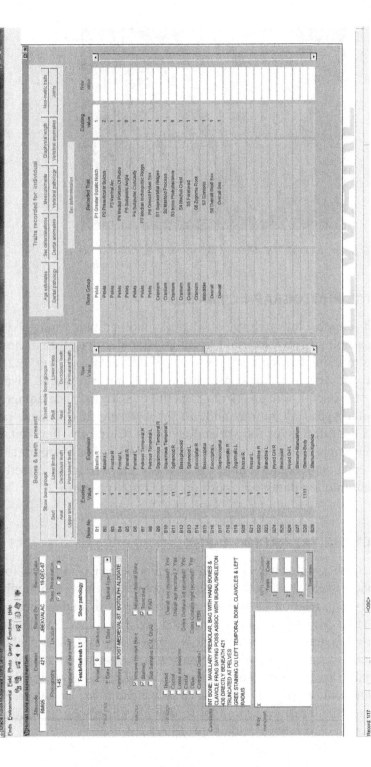

Figure 3.1 Image of database record on Wellcome Osteological Research Database (WORD), RMl05 421.

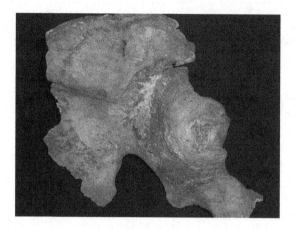

Figure 3.2 Digital photographic image (OCU00 668) healed fracture of right ilium (posterior view).

3.3 DIGITAL PHOTOGRAPHIC IMAGES

The CHB curates an archive of digital photographic images of recorded pathologies and skeletal anomalies shared in jpeg format and linked to the individual contexts on the WORD database (Fig. 3.2). This database serves as a conservation tool mitigating the over handling of skeletal remains from repetitive analysis. The images capture pathological alterations and aid in observing any changes or damage to the integrity of the skeletal elements. Currently, the digital photographic images can be viewed on the CHB website, annotated with site code and context numbers. Work is ongoing to directly upload them into the database record on the Oracle platform.

3.4 DIRECT DIGITAL RADIOGRAPHY

Previously, radiography has not been a routine aspect of analysis for archaeological skeletal collections. Radiography had more commonly been employed in relation to the study of mummies with studies such as the Manchester Mummy Project (Isherwood and Hart, 1992). Wet film radiography requires a dedicated area for processing and the variable quality of clarity, cost, problems with long-term storage, and the limited ability to share and view the wet film images are major issues (Fig. 3.3). The development of digital X-raying was considerable; as Burgener (2008) notes, "the transition from film to digital radiography has had a great impact on conventional radiology" (p. v).

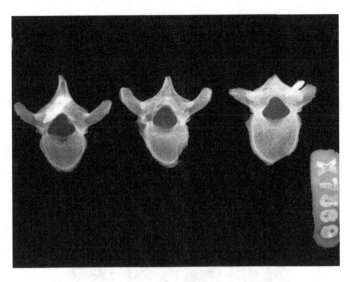

Figure 3.3 Wet film radiograph of vertebrae showing projectile injury (MIN86 5343).

Direct digital radiography (DDR) provides a rapid and relatively inexpensive means for visualizing and analyzing the internal structure of skeletal remains, revealing information otherwise impossible to access with only macroscopic analysis. The application of DDR provides important information and pathological data, allowing for an additional level of interpretation for the varying types of skeletal assemblages (Western and Bekvalac, 2015). It is nondestructive, mobile, and can produce large datasets of digital images in multiple formats that are compatible with many online platforms. The application of DDR with a radiographer enables the use of clinical protocols to be followed, aiding in the interpretation and comparison of the archaeological remains. Clinical standards and strategies in place for DICOM (Digital Imaging and Communications in Medicine) and PACS (Picture Archiving and Communication System) are well established, with protocols and standards that can be applied to the digital radiography of archaeological materials (eg, Kim et al., 2015; Müller et al., 2004; Tello et al., 2014).

Digital radiography is more versatile and has increased the opportunities for radiography to be more widely available to use on archaeological skeletal collections. DDR equipment can also be portable, which is a major advantage for skeletal remains that may be stored in difficult-to-access locations, reducing the amount of

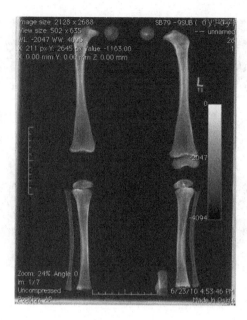

Figure 3.4 Digital radiograph of nonadult long bones of the right and left leg (SB79 9).

potential damage that may affect the remains whilst in transit. DDR has proven to be a useful tool at the CHB, with its first application to the crypt assemblage at St Bride's Church, Fleet Street, London, then to MoL collections, and excavated material from Worcester Royal Infirmary. Prof. Jerry Conlogue of Quinnipiac University, United States used a portable radiographic kit (Reveal Imaging Ltd) in the crypt at St Bride's Church, Fleet Street, establishing the basis of a burgeoning and extremely beneficial and valuable data source. The clarity of the images produced was excellent and provide another method for researching this unique biographical collection (Fig. 3.4).

The initial application of DDR to the skeletal remains retained in St Bride's crypt has already opened avenues of collaborative research (Bekvalac, 2012; Conlogue et al., in press) and more will be possible in the future when mechanisms are in place to more readily share the digital radiographic images online. DDR has also been applied as part of a number of postgraduate research projects on the curated collections at the museum, such as studies investigating growth and development in nonadults (Newman, 2015) and aiding in the identification of trauma in nonadults (Verlinden and Lewis, 2015).

Ongoing collaborative research with Gaynor Western (Ossafreelance) and Mark Farmer (Teesside University), using radiographs of female crania from St Bride's, enabled investigation into Hyperostosis Frontalis Interna (HFI) that previously would not have been possible. The results this radiographic research produced led to further research into HFI with funding in 2014 from the British Association for Biological Anthropology and Osteoarchaeology, enabling the digital radiography of 50 female crania from the Christ Church Spitalfields collection at the Natural History Museum, London, United Kingdom, with a selection of these to be scanned in a micro CT scanner (Bekvalac et al., 2014).

The newest exciting project borne of this radiographic research is "The Impact of Industrialisation on London Health." With generous funding from the City of London Archaeological Trust Rosemary Green Grant, this project is now in place for 2015–18. This project will radiograph c.2500 adults from archaeological skeletal collections in London and regional areas outside of London to expand knowledge of diseases, and address questions about the impact of urbanization on health by studying pathologies revealed from the radiographic images and macroscopic analysis. The scale of the archive will dramatically increase and the critical challenge with this developing and growing digital archive is making it accessible and maintaining it for the future. Fortunately, it is possible to store the images in a number of formats, and the clinical protocols in place with DDR used by hospitals are a good vanguard for the long-term sustainability of the digital radiographs (Western and Bekvalac, 2015).

3.5 COMPUTED TOMOGRAPHY

Medical imaging such as CT and micro CT scans are becoming increasingly available to use on osteoarchaeological material as costs decrease and access to specialist equipment becomes easier. A small number of the skeletal remains from the CHB have had CT scans, which, as with digital radiography, is a desirable nondestructive method of investigation. The CT and micro CT scans enable the skeletal remains to be viewed internally in the form of virtual slices, allowing for even greater detail than a radiograph. CT scans are made up of many radiographic images from multiple angles creating 2D images (virtual slices) that are combined in stacks to form volume data (thickness) that can be viewed in 3D. The cross-sectional images enable the skeletal elements to be viewed in sliced sections of varying thickness and provide finite details of the structure of the elements and any variations, with micro CT scanning providing a very high resolution, in the range of microns (Weber, 2015). Weber (2015) discusses the variety of imaging applications applied for creating virtual anthropology and some of the problems using them, but highlights how, with the access to such applications, the data have important implications for comparative morphology and functional analysis. CT as a method of investigation has been readily embraced in the study of mummified remains, which has led to a number of innovative research projects and exhibitions (eg, Friedman et al., 2012; Gardner et al., 2004; Nelson and Wade, 2015; Wade and Nelson, 2013; Wade et al., 2011a, 2012).

The CHB has been fortunate to have access to CT and micro CT scanners in collaboration with institutions including the Moorfields Eye Hospital, the National Hospital for Neurology and Neurosurgery, St Bartholomew's Hospital, and the Natural History Museum, London. The initial collaboration was spurred by biomedical and medical student researchers from St George's Hospital carrying out research on selected elements from the museum's skeletal collections. The students' research used the CT scanned images to aid them in investigations concerning bone density, cranial variation, and cribra orbitalia. One of these students examined two post-medieval collections at the CHB to define a protocol to be used clinically for the detection of cribra orbitalia using CT (Naveed et al., 2012). The CHB shared a CT scan of a complete skeletal individual through the exhibition *Doctors, Dissection and Resurrection Men* at the MoL in 2012–13. This was possible with access to a more sophisticated CT scanner based at The National Hospital for Neurology and Neurosurgery and the support of experienced radiologist Indran Davagnanam from Moorfields Hospital.

The size of the CT slice images can be large, which can be problematical for organizations that must ensure that they have computer systems capable of rendering the images for diagnostic interpretation and sharing. Currently the MoL does not have the computer systems, programmes, or specialist knowledge necessary to render the images for diagnostic interpretation and sharing of CT images.

3.6 3D MODELING

3D modeling is an area of developing innovation that has become increasingly popular as a beneficial interactive teaching tool. The uses of 3D modeling are found in a wide spectrum of industries, including the forensic and medical fields, with the application to archaeological and skeletal collections being more recent (eg, Gualdi-Russo et al., 2015; Szikossy et al., 2015; Woo et al., 2015). The process of 3D modeling uses specialized software, which captures the surface features of objects using a series of geometric points enabling the resultant data to be remodeled to create a virtual representation that can then be manipulated and viewed in numerous ways. As with the other digital modalities outlined, 3D modeling does have challenges and issues in its usage and application, particularly the size of the resultant dataset and the requirement for powerful computers with the necessary capacity and functionality to be able to interpret, store, and share the resultant virtual output.

The creation of a virtual 3D model has the potential for a greater tangible interaction with the skeletal collections for teaching and research while safeguarding delicate pathological lesions from over handling. The Digitised Disease Project (https://digitiseddiseases. wordpress.com/) is a groundbreaking approach to increasing access to 3D digital models of human skeletal remains with pathological lesions. A number of the individuals from the collections at the MoL were included in this project. As an integrated method of research at the CHB, 3D scans and modeling have been used in postgraduate research projects such as O'Mahoney's (2009) work concerning upper limb biomechanics using a Next Engine scanner. This model of scanner was also used by Dr. Louise Humphrey (Natural History Museum) as part of an ongoing interdisciplinary study on growth and development of nonadult skeletal remains, scanning targeted elements from the nonadult individuals from St Bride's crypt. In 2015, PhD student Rebecca Gibson (American University, Washington, DC) used a Next Engine scanner to scan ribs and vertebrae of selected adult females from St Bride's Lower Churchyard to investigate plastic thoracic deformation. Further, the virtual skeletal analysis 3D scanning project, initiated in 2012 by Roland Wessling, Dr. Sophie Beckett, and Jessica Bolton (Cranfield Forensic Institute, Cranfield University), uses 3D scanning to quantitatively investigate features of the bone surface that can otherwise only be observed qualitatively.

3.7 DISCUSSION

The opportunity to apply digital techniques to archaeological collections, notably skeletal remains, has provided remarkable means of storing, generating, engaging, interacting with, and interpreting extensive datasets. The CHB digital archive is already extensive and will continue to develop and grow. The osteological database is a powerful digital asset and has already proved to be the most invaluable research tool for integrated research. Working alongside radiographers, radiologists, and specialists in the digital imaging fields has been particularly important with the application of digital radiography integrated as a research tool for projects in the CHB.

The application of the digital imaging techniques discussed in this paper allows for the study of the MoL collections from multiple angles. Integration of the datasets can provide a more extensive yet nuanced understanding of the skeletal collections. The data provided from each technique are unique, thus the application of multiple modalities encourages the examination of research questions from many angles and increases not only the amount of information gained, but the strength of the evidence. Where digital photographs and 3D modeling provide detailed information on exterior structures of bone, digital radiographs and CT scans provide increasingly detailed information on internal morphology and microarchitecture. Combining, for example, radiographs and CT can be used to explore pathological changes (Wade et al., 2011b). Similarly, 3D modeling and radiographs or CT can be used to correlate exterior surface changes with interior morphological differences. Having this information accessible for researchers at the MoL allows for the creation of more complex research questions and more detailed answers that push the field of osteology forward. Use of these technologies does, however, require acknowledging their limitations in order to integrate them appropriately.

The next step for the CHB is to actively promote the use of integrated modalities in the research conducted at the Centre. For example the large-scale City of London Archaeological Trust (CoLAT) funded project, "The Impact of Industrialisation on London Health" will be the first project for the Centre that will be able to fully utilize all of the imaging modalities to address a particular research question. This project is intended as a large-scale investigation of the changing health patterns of medieval and post-medieval London, with specific attention to the role that industrialization played. For this project, uniting the multiple modalities is key to establishing a cohesive overview of change in general health patterns as it allows for examination of a wider range of indicators than would be accessible with any one method, and that together speak to larger shifts in human health.

There are enormous positive attributes to digital applications, but they have their associated challenges. Digital systems can develop rapidly and heritage institutions are under increasing financial pressures; thus, maintaining and updating digital assets can be difficult. Maintaining the integrity of and long-term access to digital records will continue to be a challenge. The security of data, server capacity, and back up for data are vital for the integrity of the data and long-term storage. The sustainability of digital archives requires the maintenance of systems and functionality, the prevention and management of the degradation of digital data formats, and support for digital assets and training.

Questions about standards and best practices in light of digital resources and access have recently been raised (Atkin, 2015) and a working group has been proposed to discuss the ethical implications of sharing digital images of human remains. Standards and codes of ethics exist for many aspects relating to human remains (eg, Historic England, 2005; British Association for Biological Anthropology and Osteoarchaeology, 2010; Department for Culture, Media and Sport, 2005), but such codes are often virtually nonexistent with digital resources. These challenges will continue to be an issue as digital technologies develop and images relating to human remains reach wider audiences.

Digital applications enhance the knowledge we can glean from the people of the past, open up channels of information, and have the potential to forge global interdisciplinary relationships for learning, but the applications themselves cannot replace the actual skeletal remains. The CHB firmly believes that the retention and curation of the physical remains is paramount and that the digital applications are a means of fully amplifying the bioarchaeological information, the "voice of the past" from the skeletons (Larsen, 2002, p. 3). Expectations of the providers and users have been completely altered by advancing digital technologies and provide access to untold treasures of information about the past. Managing that access can be problematic, but the CHB is an example of an institution where digital applications have been able to open up access to a unique archive, are an invaluable asset, and continue to share data on a scale that would have once been thought impossible.

REFERENCES

Atkin, A., 2015. Digging the digital dead. In: 17th Annual Conference of the British Association for Biological Anthropology and Osteoarchaeology, University of Sheffield, paper presentation.

Bekvalac, J., 2012. Implementation of preliminary digital radiographic examination in the confines of the crypt of St Bride's Church, Fleet Street, London. In: Proceedings of the Twelfth Annual Conference of the British Association for Biological Anthropology and Osteoarchaeology. BAR International Series 2380, 111–118.

Bekvalac, J., Western, G., Farmer, M., 2014. The impact of industrialisation on female health: understanding the aetiology of hyperostosis frontalis interna. In: 16th Annual Conference of the British Association for Biological Anthropology and Osteoarchaeology, University of Durham, poster presentation.

Brickley, M., McKinley, J., 2004. Guidelines to the standards for recording human remains. British Association for Biological Anthropology and Osteoarchaeology and Institute of Field Archaeologists. Available online: <http://www.babao.org.uk/HumanremainsFINAL.pdf>.

British Association for Biological Anthropology and Osteoarchaeology, 2010. Code of Ethics. Available online: <http://www.babao.org.uk/index/cms-filesystem-action/code%20of%20ethics.pdf>.

Buikstra, J.E., Ubelaker, D.H. (Eds.), 1994. Standards for Data Collection from Human Skeletal Remains. Arkansas Archaeological Survey, Research Series No. 44. Fayetteville, Arkansas.

Burgener, A.F., 2008. Preface. In: Burgener, A.F., Kormano, M., Pudas, T. (Eds.), Bone and Joint Disorders. Differential Diagnosis in Conventional Radiology, 3rd ed. George Thieme Verlag, Stuttgart, p. v.

Conlogue, G., Viner, V., Beckett, R., Bekvalac, J., Gonzalez, R., Sharkey, M., et al., 2016. A post-mortem evaluation of the degree of mobility in an individual with severe kyphoscoliosis using direct digital radiography (DDR) and multi-detector computed tomography (MDCT). In: Tilley, L., Schrenk, A. (Eds.), New Developments in the Bioarchaeology of Care: Further Case Studies and Extended Theory. Springer, New York (Chapter 7).

Connell, B., Rauxloh, P., 2003. A Rapid Method for Recording Human Skeletal Data. Museum of London Report, London.

Connell, B., Gray Jones, A., Redfern, R., Walker, D., 2012. A Bioarchaeological Study of Medieval Burials on the Site of St Mary Spital: Excavations at Spitalfields Market, London E1, 1991–2007. MoLA Monograph Series 60.

Department for Culture, Media and Sport, 2005. Guidance on the Care of Human Remains in Museums. London. Available online: <http://www.babao.org.uk/index/cms-filesystem-action?file=dcmsguide%20oct%202005.pdf>.

Friedman, S.N., Nguyen, N., Nelson, A.J., Granton, P.V., MacDonald, D.B., Hibbert, R., et al., 2012. Computed tomography (CT) bone segmentation of an ancient Egyptian mummy: a comparison of automated and semiautomated threshold and dual-energy techniques. J. Comput. Assist. Tomogr. 36, 616–622.

Gardner, J.C., Garvin, G., Nelson, A.J., Vascotto, G., Conlogue, G., 2004. Paleoradiology in mummy studies: the Sulman mummy project. Can. Assoc. Radiol. J. 55, 228–234.

Gualdi-Russo, E., Zaccagni, L., Russo, V., 2015. Giovanni Battista Morgagni: facial reconstruction by virtual anthropology. Forensic Sci. Med. Pathol. 11, 222–227.

Historic England, 2005. Guidance for best practice for treatment of human remains excavated from Christian burial grounds in England. Available online: <https://content.historicengland.org.uk/images-books/publications/human-remains-excavated-from-christian-burial-grounds-in-england/16602humanremains1.pdf/>.

Isherwood, I., Hart, C.W., 1992. The radiological investigation. In: David, A.R., Tapp, E. (Eds.), The Mummy's Tale. Michael O'Mara Books, London, pp. 100–111.

Kim, T., Heo, E., Lee, M., Kim, J., Yoo, S., Kim, S., et al., 2015. Medical image exchange and sharing between heterogeneous picture archiving and communication systems based upon international standard: pilot implantation. 15th International HL7 Interoperability Conference Proceedings, 37–42 <http://ihic2015.hl7cr.eu/Proceedings-web.pdf>.

Larsen, C.S., 2002. Skeletons in Our Closet: Revealing Our Past through Bioarchaeology. Princeton University Press, Princeton.

Müller, H., Michoux, N., Bandon, D., Geissbuhler, A., 2004. A review of content-based image retrieval systems in medical applications—clinical benefits and future directions. Int. J. Med. Inform. 73, 1–23.

Naveed, H., Abed, S.F., Davagnanam, I., Uddin, J.M., Adds, P.J., 2012. Lessons from the past: cribra orbitalia, an orbital roof pathology. Orbit 31, 394–399.

Nelson, A.J., Wade, A.D., 2015. Impact: development of a radiological mummy database. Anat. Rec. 298, 941–948.

Newman, S., 2015. The growth of a nation: child health and development in the industrial revolution in England, c. AD 1750–1850. Durham University, Department of Archaeology, Durham (unpublished PhD thesis).

O'Mahoney, T., 2009. Activity and allometry: a three dimensional study of humeri from contrasting populations using three dimensional laser scans. University College London, London (unpublished MSc dissertation).

Powers, N. (Ed.), 2012. Human Osteology Method Statement. Museum of London Report, London. Available: <http://archive.museumoflondon.org.uk/NR/rdonlyres/3A7B0C25-FD36-4D43-863E-B2FDC5A86FB7/0/OsteologyMethodStatementrevised2012.pdf>.

Roberts, C., Mays, S., 2011. Study and restudy of curated skeletal collections in bioarchaeology: a perspective on the UK and the implications for future curation of human remains. Int. J. Osteoarchaeol. 21, 626–630.

Szikossy, I., Pálfi, G., Molnár, E., Karlinger, K., Kovács, B.K., Korom, C., et al., 2015. Two positive tuberculosis cases in the late Nigrovits family, 18th century, Vác, Hungary. Tuberculosis 95 (S1), S69–S72.

Tello, A., La Cruz, A., Saquicela, V., Espinoza, M., Vidal, M.-E., 2014. RDF-ization of DICOM medical images towards linked health data cloud. IFMBE Proc. 49, 757–760.

Thomas, C., 2004. Life and Death in London's East End: 2000 Years at Spitalfields. MoLAS, London.

Verlinden, P., Lewis, M.E., 2015. Childhood trauma: methods for the identification of physeal fractures in nonadult skeletal remains. Am. J. Phys. Anthropol. 157, 411–420.

Wade, A.D., Nelson, A.J., 2013. Radiological evaluation of the evisceration tradition in ancient Egyptian mummies. Homo 64, 1–28.

Wade, A.D., Nelson, A.J., Garvin, G.J., 2011a. A synthetic radiological study of brain treatment in ancient Egyptian mummies. Homo 62, 248–269.

Wade, A.D., Holdsworth, D.W., Garvin, G.J., 2011b. CT and micro-CT analysis of a case of Paget's disease (osteitis deformans) in the Grant skeletal collection. Int. J. Osteoarch 21, 127–135.

Wade, A.D., Garvin, G.J., Hurnanen, J.H., Williams, L.L., Lawson, B., Nelson, A.J., et al., 2012. Scenes from the past: multidetector CT of Egyptian mummies of the Redpath Museum. Radiographics 32, 1235–1250.

Weber, G.W., 2015. Virtual anthropology. Yearb. Phys. Anthropol. 156, 22–42.

Western, A.G., Bekvalac, J., 2015. Digital radiography and historical contextualisation of the 19th century modified human skeletal remains from the Worcester Royal Infirmary, England. Int. J. Palaeopath. 10, 58–73.

Woo, E.J., Lee, W.-J., Hu, K.-S., Hwang, J.J., 2015. Paleopathological study of dwarfism-related skeletal dysplasia in a late Joseon dynasty (South Korean) population. PLoS One 10, e0140901. Available from: http://dx.doi.org/10.1371/journal.pone.0140901.

CHAPTER 4

"Readmitted Under Urgent Circumstance": Uniting Archives and Bioarchaeology at the Royal London Hospital

M. Mant
Department of Anthropology, McMaster University, Hamilton, ON, Canada

4.1 INTRODUCTION

Contemporary documentary evidence is of immense value in historical bioarchaeological studies. There are, however, limitations and challenges inherent in the use of past records that must be addressed. The Royal London Hospital, a voluntary hospital founded in 1740 in London, United Kingdom, provides an engaging case study in which multiple lines of evidence are examined to investigate the frequency of fractures during the mid-18th to early 19th centuries (c.1760–1805). Both the skeletal remains of individuals who were admitted to, and subsequently died in, the hospital, and a limited set of hospital admission records are extant. This study addresses the key query: what body areas did the working poor, admitted to the Royal London Hospital, fracture most frequently? Hospital admission records provide one dataset, while the bones of individuals excavated from 18th-century and early 19th-century burial grounds provide another.

This paper explores how the archival and human skeletal remain datasets, in spite of their biases and limitations, intersect to provide a complex view of fractures and medical intervention in 18th- and early 19th-century London (Fig. 4.1).

4.2 THE ROYAL LONDON HOSPITAL

The 18th century has been referred to as the Age of Hospitals in reference to the expansion of medical care during this period (Dainton, 1961). Enlightenment ideals encouraged charitable giving

Beyond the Bones. DOI: http://dx.doi.org/10.1016/B978-0-12-804601-2.00004-1

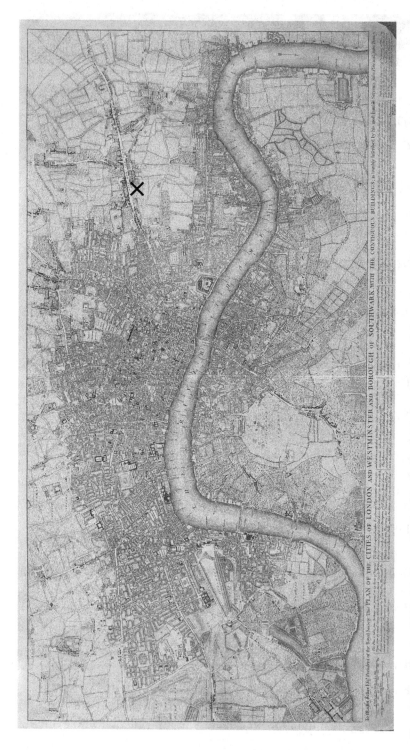

Figure 4.1 Map of London, 1746 by John Rocque. The Royal London Hospital site is marked with an X. Source: Image © Museum of London.

and London became a focus of charity since it was a place where "the middle and professional classes were particularly in evidence, where funds were most easily gathered, and where social problems were most visible" (Levene, 2006, p. xiii; Langford, 1989). The Royal London Hospital, founded in 1740, located on Whitechapel Road, was one of four voluntary hospitals operating in London during the 18th century, institutions dependent upon donations, subscriptions, and fund-raising events to provide charitable care for London's poor. The hospital received its royal designation in 1990 at its 250th anniversary. The voluntary hospitals were founded upon "a wave of philanthropy by those who wished not merely to alleviate distress but to restore the afflicted to respectable and independent citizenhood" (Rivett, 1986, p. 25). These hospitals were designed to care for the working poor, a group that depended upon wage labor and could not afford to pay for their medical treatment (Dyson, 2014). The Royal London Hospital, in particular, was likely to admit a large number of accident cases due to its location, "which is placed in the centre of one of the densest and poorest districts, and in close proximity to the Docks" (Bristowe and Holmes, qtd. in Woodward, 1974, p. 130).

Generally patients were admitted once each week; however, accident cases were admitted at any time (Clark-Kennedy, 1962). Prospective patients were required to obtain a letter of recommendation by a hospital governor, an individual who had given a charitable donation to the hospital and was thereby given the right to recommend a certain number of individuals for hospital admission (Howard, 1791; Lawrence, 1996). If an individual died in hospital and friends or family did not retrieve their body, they would be buried at the hospital's expense.

4.2.1 Dataset Challenges: Age Estimation

The ages recorded or estimated in the two datasets, the skeletal remains and archival records, have different implications. In skeletal studies the estimated age is the individual's age at death, whereas the hospital records provide information on the chronological age of an individual when they arrived at the hospital with a fracture. Age-specific rates for nonfatal antemortem fractures are impossible to calculate (Waldron, 1991) since it is unclear at what age a fracture was incurred. Fractures observed in a skeleton reflect the cumulative number of fractures acquired over the individual's lifetime.

Age estimation limitations are a chronic plague upon bioarchaeological studies. The ability to correlate osteological and clinical data is hindered by this challenge (Glencross, 2011; Glencross and Sawchuk, 2003) and much attention has been paid to exploring the limitations in determining age distributions from skeletal samples (eg, Hoppa and Vaupel, 2002). The broad age categories used in skeletal studies are necessary since aging adult individuals involves the imprecise categorization of macroscopic degenerative changes present in the skeleton. Chronological age in the hospital records is more easily accessible. If a patient's age was not recorded, the categories were even broader than those of skeletal estimations: an individual could only be labeled as a juvenile, an adult, or unknown. When the age of the patient was listed; however, the hospital admissions dataset offers exactitude that a skeletal dataset cannot approach.

4.2.2 Dataset Challenges: Human Error and Representation in Documentary Sources

The largest limitation in consulting archival records, as referenced above, is that the data collected are limited to which records have survived and are available for study. As Chodorow wryly observed, "the cultural record will be just what got saved because someone put it in a safe place" (2006, p. 373). Further, the hospital admissions do not record which side a fractured element came from or the location of the fracture on the bone. This fact complicates the possible comparisons to be made with the skeletal data. For example, a "fractured humerus" found in the archival records could be an antemortem fracture inferior of the surgical neck of the left humerus or a crush fracture of the right olecranon fossa, but that level of detail is simply unattainable in the admissions records. This lack of detail in the hospital admission records necessitates the use of broad anatomical groupings when seeking to investigate meaningful comparisons with the skeletal data.

Fowler and Powers (2012a), in their elegant study of the excavation of the Royal London Burial Ground by Museum of London Archaeology, note that no admission registers exist for the temporal period matching the dates of the burials; this limitation complicates any attempt to compare the records and remains from a single site. The authors employ the 1841 census to provide a "snapshot" of patients that were in the London Hospital on Jun. 6, 1841. In the present case, the extant hospital admission registers are utilized as part of an exercise to illustrate the potential rewards and inherent limitations of drawing upon multiple lines of evidence to approach a historical research question.

Humans make mistakes. Risse (1986) details how the expansion and consequent increased registration at the Royal Infirmary of Edinburgh caused the hospital clerks to become overwhelmed. Certain admission papers went missing or information was not transferred due to the clerks having "too much business" (Royal Infirmary of Edinburgh, Minute Books, Vol. 4, 1770, p. 227). Grauer characterizes human record keeping as "overwhelmingly erratic" (1995, p. ix). Allowing adequate time to untangle the threads of historical documentation is key to catching possible errors. Mitchell (2012) emphasizes the importance of studying primary documents to understand "who wrote them, why they were written, for whom they were written, and exactly when they were written" (p. 316). Thankfully, the motivation of hospital record keepers is clear and the documents consulted in this research were dated. Reasonable expectations for how accurately historical documentation reflects historical reality are necessary. Various authors have characterized the historian or user of the archives as a detective (eg, Ginzburg, 1989; Winks, 1969), emphasizing that the "probative value of evidence in a particular setting" (Turkel, 2006, p. 260) requires careful reflection.

There are limitations to both historical and contemporary clinical reports concerning fracture frequencies; primarily, individuals admitted to hospital are self-selecting (eg, Court-Brown and Caesar, 2006; Koval and Cooley, 2006; Lane, 2001). There have been valiant attempts to quantify the commonness of different fractures through analyses of modern hospital data from the United Kingdom (eg, Buhr and Cooke, 1959; Court-Brown and Caesar, 2006; Singer et al., 1998), but ultimately the data depend upon individuals choosing to seek medical attention. In addition, data are derived from particular hospitals, ensuring that the results are geographically specific (eg, Donaldson et al., 1990; Johansen et al., 1997; Sahlin, 1990; van Staa et al., 2001). The same was true in London during the 18th and early 19th centuries. Admission was complicated by a variety of unfamiliar factors to a modern observer, such as official admissions being allowed only once a week in certain institutions, and the necessity of campaigning for a hospital governor's permission for admittance (Carruthers and Carruthers, 2005; Dainton, 1961; Lane, 2001; Lawrence, 1996).

4.2.3 Diagnostic Labels: A Paean for Fractures as a Connection to the Past

Ensuring that terms are clearly defined aids in the comparative use of skeletal and documentary data (eg, Howell, 1986; Petersen, 1975). Risse (1986) refers to physicians' diagnoses as diagnostic labels, or reasons for admission/death as medical practitioners understood them at the time. Rosenberg and Golden (1992) and Cunningham (2002) among others (eg, Arrizabalaga, 2002; Hays, 2007; Metcalfe, 2007; Mitchell, 2011) discuss the complex nature of studying disease in the past; one must consider the modern biological diagnosis and the social diagnosis used by individuals in the past. Information gleaned from surgeons' casebooks and the catalogues of contemporary anatomical collections suggests that surgeons had an understanding of fracture causes and treatments that is comparable to modern understandings. Eighteenth-century physicians conceived of disease diagnoses as a form of taxonomy including classes, orders, genera, and species, following the example of botanists (King, 1958). Fractures, according to William Cullen (1792), were defined as "bones broken into large fragments" (p. 80). This definition is similar to both current clinical and palaeo-pathological definitions of fracture, suggesting that fractures are reasons for hospital admission that transcend time more easily than, for example, diagnoses of "foul" diseases that may encompass many venereal complaints or conditions that are unfamiliar to modern eyes, such as St Vitus's Dance.

Medical students during the 18th century were certainly exposed to education concerning fractures. A surgical student at St Thomas' Hospital recorded in his notebook, covering the years 1725 and 1726, detailed descriptions of the causes and treatments of cranial, femoral, tibial, and fibular fractures (King's College London, 1725–1726, GB 0100 TH/PP44). An indirect source of evidence suggesting that physicians and surgeons at the voluntary hospitals would be well-versed in the appearance of fractures are the pathological collections at institutions such as St Bartholomew's and Westminster hospitals and the Royal College of Surgeons. The Westminster Hospital pathology collection, which was started in the 18th century, was 39% comprised of fracture specimens by the 19th century (19/49 total specimens) (Mitchell and Chauhan, 2012, p. 143). Mitchell and Chauhan (2012) posit that the proportion of specimens representing fractures may be so high because surgeons thought they were particularly important, or perhaps fractures were among the most common conditions affecting bone at the time. Another possibility is that fractures were relatively simple to observe and identify in living patients (Mitchell and Chauhan, 2012) and that surgeons were curious to observe fractures at various stages of healing. Almost exactly half of the Royal College of Surgeons anatomy and pathology collection (pre-1886) were fracture specimens (1016/2036 = 49.9%). The St Bartholomew's Anatomical Museum descriptive catalogue (Paget, 1846) includes over 200 descriptions of fracture specimens, ranging from relatively minor metacarpal fractures to devastating long bone and skull fractures. Many specimens are healed antemortem fractures, and include patient histories, such as a male individual who suffered a midshaft humeral fracture four years before death. He was "so little impaired by the fracture that [he] worked as a sailor to the time of his death" (1846, p. 116). These sources of evidence suggest that fractures were a relatively common sight in medical education and that a diagnosis of "fracture" or "broken" accurately refers to a broken bone.

4.3 MATERIALS AND METHODS: RECORDS AND REMAINS

4.3.1 Hospital Admission Records

Hospital admission books have survived from 1760, 1791, 1792, and the latter half of 1805 and are curated by the Royal London Hospital Museum. The records note the name, date of admittance, place of abode, occupation, age, reason for admission, and result of hospital stay for each individual. Sex of the admitted individuals was determined through examination of their given names. Additional clues to an individual's sex were provided under the occupation column, since many women were recorded as being a "Sailors Wife," "Labourers Wife," or a "Washerwoman." Individuals for whom sex could not be confidently assigned were removed from the final study sample. The records for 1760, 1791, and 1792 list the age of the admitted individual. Whipple's index (Siegel and Swanson, 2004) was calculated for this sample and found to be 167.9 for the male sample and 167.3 for the females. Whipple's index is a summary index calculated by taking the sum of the number of individuals reporting their age as 25, 30, 35, 40, 45, 50, 55, and 60, multiplying this total by 5, dividing the result by the number of individuals in the age categories 23−62 inclusive and multiplying the result by 100. An index below 105 indicates that the dataset is highly accurate, between 105−110 the data are relatively accurate, 110—125 the data are approximate, 125—175 the data are poor, and 175+ the data are very poor (United Nations, 1955; Newell, 1988). Individuals in the past often did not know their exact age and estimated when asked, meaning that ages ending with zero or five were more likely to be stated and recorded. The Whipple results indicate that there is a substantial inaccuracy in the reporting of ages.

This research was conducted exclusively on adult individuals; an adult was defined as an individual aged 18 years or older. Adults were chosen as the focus in order to make meaningful comparisons between the skeletal findings and contemporary archival evidence of hospital admissions. Though children do appear in the archival hospital records, it is overwhelmingly adult individuals who received treatment at London's voluntary hospitals. Skeletal sex estimation techniques do not allow for confident sex estimations to be made for individuals under about 18 years of age. Further, adults would have been responsible for securing their own admission (Risse, 1986; Wilde, 1810) or that of their family members.

A total of 3703 individuals formed the study sample from the London hospital admission registers: 2285 males and 1418 females. Age was recorded for 3160 of these individuals, 1910 males and 1250 females. The ages of the admitted individuals are displayed in Table 4.1 and Fig. 4.2 by decade; the majority of records fall in the 18- to 30-year-old category (38.0% of males and 48.5% of females) with the number of admissions decreasing in the upper age categories. Fisher's Exact Test was performed to compare the number of male and female admissions by age category; there is a statistically significant ($p < 0.0001$) larger proportion of females in the 18—30 age group and males in the 31—40 age group.

Table 4.1 Age Distribution of Individuals in Hospital Admission Records by Sex		
Age Category	Males	Females
18—30	726 (38.0)	606 (48.5)
31—40	519 (27.2)	230 (18.4)
41—50	345 (18.1)	241 (19.3)
51—60	215 (11.3)	119 (9.5)
61—70	85 (4.5)	40 (3.2)
71—80	14 (0.7)	13 (1.0)
81—90	6 (0.3)	1 (0.1)
Total	1910	1250

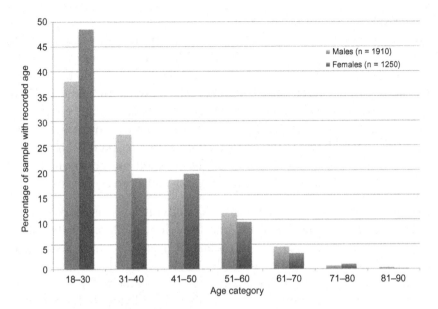

Figure 4.2 Age distribution of adult individuals in hospital admission records.

When assessing the reasons for admission, entries that stated an individual had a "fracture" or a "broken" body element were counted as fractures, while elements that were recorded as "bruised," "hurt," or "injured" were disregarded. It is possible that an individual may have been admitted to hospital with an injury that appeared as a bruise or laceration but was actually a fracture; therefore, the fracture frequencies reported may underestimate the number of fractures treated in the voluntary hospitals.

To assess the quality of the archival dataset, Michael Drake's (1982, p. vii) algorithm concerning English parish records was adopted. Drake (1982) examines the quality and reliability of vital record datasets (eg, birth, death, and marriage certificates) to aid the researcher in deciding which records to consult. The present research sample fulfills Drake's (1982) criteria for acceptable data quality: the admission records contain more than 100 entries per year, there is no obvious evidence of underregistration in the records, and the gaps present in the records are not a deterrent since the case study aims to explore the potential limitations of engaging with multiple datasets rather than investigating temporal trends in hospital fracture registration.

4.3.2 Human Skeletal Remains

Individuals from the Royal London Hospital burial ground are curated at the Museum of London Centre for Human Bioarchaeology under the site code RLP05. The 2006 excavation by Museum of London Archaeology uncovered burials dating from between 1825 and 1841. In addition to individuals in standard wooden coffins, burials comprising skeletal elements from multiple individuals were also discovered, many of which showed evidence of autopsy or anatomization. Graves generally contained between one and five stacked burials, though there were outliers with as many as eight (Fowler and Powers, 2012b).

Individuals were selected for this study if at least 30% of the skeleton was present. The Wellcome Osteological Research Database (WORD) maintained by the Museum of London was consulted to determine how many adult individuals of greater than 30% skeletal completeness were present. The aim was to exclude as few individuals as possible while minimizing the number of individuals for whom it would be impossible to assess sex and estimate age due to poor overall completeness. A total of 110 individuals, 80 males and 30 females, formed the final study sample.

Individuals were assessed for sex by examining the skeletal remains macroscopically following the example set by Buikstra and Ubelaker (1994). Individuals were assigned to one of five categories: male, probable male, undetermined, probable female, and female. Individuals in the probable categories were combined with the male and female categories and the adults of indeterminate sex were removed from the final study sample. Age was estimated by examining four features of specific areas of the skeleton: the pubic symphysis (Brooks and Suchey, 1990), the auricular surface of the ilium (Lovejoy et al., 1985), the sternal end of ribs (Isçan and Loth, 1986a,b), and tooth wear (Brothwell, 1981). Individuals were assigned to one of five age categories, based upon those outlined by Powers (2012): young adult (18−25 years old); middle adult 1 (26−35 years old); middle adult 2 (36−45 years old); old adult (46+ years old); and adult (18+ years old). These categories were employed to allow for interobserver comparisons to be made between age estimations and those recorded in the WORD by Museum of London Archaeology observers. The age distribution of the skeletal sample is displayed in Table 4.2 and Fig. 4.3. The largest proportions of the sample were assigned to the two middle adult age

Table 4.2 Number of Individuals in Skeletal Sample Organized by Age Category and Sex		
Age Category (Years Old)	Males	Females
18−25	8 (10.0)	5 (16.7)
26−35	23 (28.8)	10 (33.3)
36−45	27 (33.8)	9 (30.0)
46 +	9 (11.3)	3 (10.0)
Adult	13 (16.3)	3 (10.0)
Total	80	30

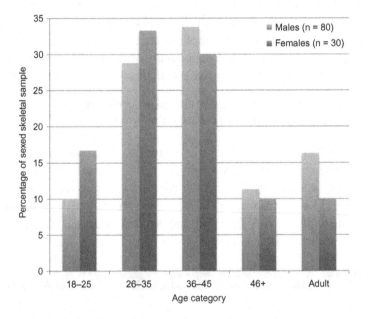

Figure 4.3 Age distribution of adult individuals in skeletal sample.

categories in both the males (28.8% and 33.8%) and females (33.3% and 30.0%). There were no statistically significant differences found between the male and female groups for any age category.

Fractures were observed macroscopically and with the aid of a Keyence VHX-2000 digital microscope. The location (by bone segment), stage of healing, and, where possible, the angle of injury were recorded. It was not possible to X-ray the remains; therefore, assertion of the angle of injury was only made when the fracture line was clearly observable macroscopically or there were radiographs available from previous studies. All observed fractures were recorded and the total number of elements present was noted. For the purposes of this case study involving affected elements, the antemortem and perimortem fracture results were combined.

4.4 RESULTS

The overall crude prevalence of individuals with one or more fractures is displayed in Table 4.3 by sex. A chi-square test was performed, revealing no significant difference between the datasets (chi-square statistic 2.9117, p-value: 0.087941, $p < 0.05$). Males make up a higher proportion of the individuals with fractures in both the hospital admission records and the skeletal sample, differences which were significant in both the records at $p < 0.05$ (chi-square statistic: 32.9061, p-value: 0) and the skeletal datasets (chi-square statistic: 8.5482, p-value: 0).

The bones were divided into anatomical groups in order to compare the two datasets, as outlined in Table 4.4.

Figs. 4.4 and 4.5 display the fracture data as proportions of the total number of fractures observed in the skeletal sample or admitted to hospital. A z-test for two proportions was performed upon these data. The proportion of skull, torso, hand, and foot fractures is significantly higher ($p < 0.05$) in the skeletal dataset for the males, while the admission records have a significant higher proportion

Table 4.3 Number of Individuals With Fractures by Sex and Dataset			
Dataset	Male n (%)	Female n (%)	Total
Records	275 (74.1)	96 (25.9)	371
Skeletons	49 (84.5)	9 (15.5)	58

Table 4.4 Anatomical Groups for Dataset Comparison	
Anatomical Group	Skeletal Elements
Skull	Cranium, facial skeleton, mandible
Torso	Sternum, ribs, vertebrae, sacrum, os coxae
Arm	Scapula, clavicle, humerus, radius, ulna
Hand	Carpals, metacarpals, manual phalanges
Leg	Femur, tibia, fibula, patella
Foot	Tarsals, metatarsals, pedal phalanges

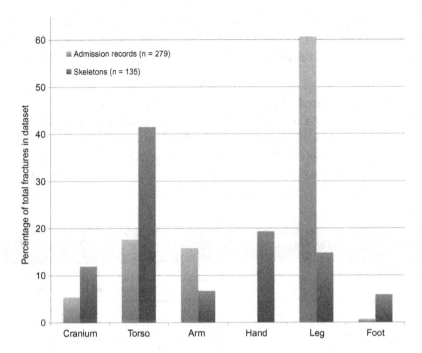

Figure 4.4 Male fracture distribution by anatomical group in skeletal and admission record datasets.

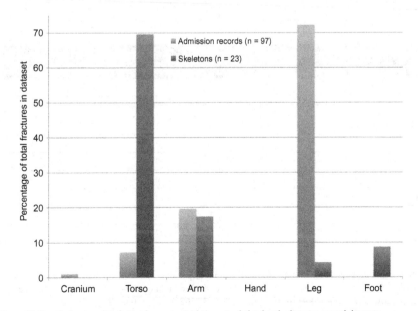

Figure 4.5 Female fracture distribution by anatomical group in skeletal and admission record datasets.

of arm and leg fractures recorded.[1] The female group showed a significantly higher proportion of torso fractures in the skeletal sample, and a significantly higher proportion of leg fractures in the admission records.[2]

The frequency of the fractured elements, grouped into anatomical areas, was compared between the two datasets for each sex and the results are displayed in Tables 4.5 and 4.6. Spearman's rank-order correlation was calculated for the data in Tables 4.5 and 4.6. The r_s value for Table 4.5 was 0.0429, indicating a weak positive correlation between the male and female datasets. The r_s value for Table 4.6 was 0.9286, indicating a strong positive correlation between the male and

Table 4.5 Rank Orders of Fractures by Sex and Anatomical Group in the Skeletal Dataset				
Anatomical Group	Males		Females	
	#Fractured Elements	Rank	# Fractured Elements	Rank
Skull	16	4	0	5
Torso	56	1	16	1
Arm	9	5	4	2
Hand	26	2	0	5
Leg	20	3	1	4
Foot	8	6	2	3
Total	135		23	

Table 4.6 Rank Order of Fractures by Sex and Anatomical Element in the Admission Records				
Anatomical Group	Males		Females	
	#Fractured Elements	Rank	# Fractured Elements	Rank
Skull	15	4	1	4
Torso	49	2	7	3
Arm	44	3	19	2
Hand	0	6	0	5
Leg	169	1	70	1
Foot	2	5	0	5
Total	279		97	

[1]Male significant z-scores: Skull (z-score: −2.3466, p-value: 0.01878), Torso (z-score: −5.2437, p-value: 0), Arm (z-score: 2.599, p-value: 0.00932), Hand (z-score: −7.5719, p-value: 0), Leg (z-score: 8.7623, p-value: 0), Foot (z-score: −3.2362, p-value: 0.0012).
[2]Female z-scores: Torso (z-score: −6.83, p-value: 0), Leg (z-score: 5.9491, p-value: 0).

female datasets. These results suggest that the relationship between the reasons for which males and females were seeking admission to the hospital is stronger than the relationship between the types of fractures observed in the skeletal datasets.

The ages of individuals admitted to the Royal London Hospital with the three most frequently fractured categories (leg, arm, and torso/ribs) from 1760, 1791, and 1792 are displayed graphically in Figs. 4.6 and 4.7 divided by age category. In the male sample, leg

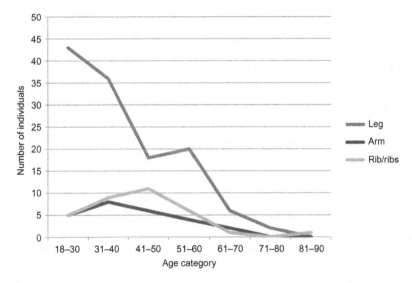

Figure 4.6 Most frequently fractured anatomical groups in male admission record sample over time.

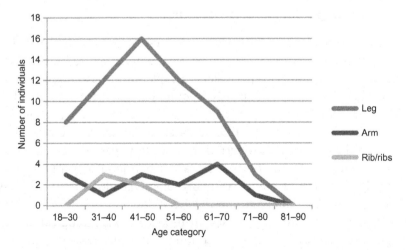

Figure 4.7 Most frequently fractured anatomical groups in female admission record sample over time.

fractures (including admissions for leg, thigh/femur, and knee/patella fractures) are the most frequent in the 18–30 age category; the admissions drop from age 31 to 50 and increase slightly in the 51–60 age group before dropping with increasing age. In contrast, the female leg fracture admissions steadily increase from age 18 to 50 before dropping off in frequency with increasing age.

4.5 DISCUSSION

It is evident that fractures to elements of the leg are common in both sexes in the admissions record, but are underrepresented in the skeletal sample. Simple sampling bias may be the culprit; the small skeletal sample may not be representative of the individuals profiled in the admission records. The ultimate fate of individuals suffering leg fractures also has an impact on these results. Individuals who successfully convalesced and were discharged from hospital, or those who died and were claimed by family or friends would not be buried at the Royal London Hospital. In addition, individuals who died in hospital during the period under investigation may have been subjected to autopsy and anatomization (Chamberlain, 2012; Chaplin, 2012; Mitchell et al., 2011). Mitchell and Chauhan (2012) posit that conditions such as severe fractures would have been relatively simple to identify in living patients; surgeons, therefore may have chosen in advance of an individual's death to include a particular anatomical specimen in the collection. There is ample evidence for anatomization at the London Hospital (Fowler and Powers, 2012b) such as "non-survivable interventions" (p. 90), including perimortem craniotomies.

The common nature of rib fractures is clear from both the skeletal and archival data. Ribs are the most frequently fractured element for both males and females in the skeletal sample; in the admissions sample ribs are the fourth most frequently fractured element for males and the fifth for the female sample. Roberts and Cox (2003) compiled data on 32,865 individuals from 201 different archaeological sites covering the Roman to the post-medieval period. In each time period (Roman, early medieval, late medieval, post-medieval), rib fractures were the most frequently fractured element. As many bioarchaeological studies have noted (eg, Brickley, 2006; Jurmain, 1999; Warden et al., 2002), underreporting of rib fractures is an issue in modern epidemiological studies, though rib fractures are the most common clinically reported injury to the thorax (Kramaker and Anthony, 2003; Tekinbas et al., 2003) and clinical studies have revealed that even a single rib fracture can cause enough pain to lower an individual's quality of life and affect their ability to work (Kara et al., 2003). The datasets each have strengths: the skeletal data provides more detail on the location and side of the fracture, which may provide clues as to the etiology of the injury, while the archival data provide a tighter age estimate for individuals suffering a rib fracture. Rib fractures are described in surgeons' notebooks from the mid-18th to early 19th centuries as a common injury. Benjamin Brodie, surgeon at St. George's Hospital, noted that "the yielding motion of the ribs prevents their being fractured so often as they would else be, but from their being so much exposed to injury, the fracture is nevertheless very frequent" (1805–1807, no page number). Patients admitted to hospital with rib fractures would be treated with "a bandage, passed several times round the thorax, so as to compress the ribs, and prevent their motion in respiration" (Brodie, 1805–1807, no page number). This simple remedy could be effected in the home, possibly explaining why the proportion of rib fractures in the skeletal sample was significantly higher than that in the admission results.

The fractures observed frequently in the skeletal sample, such as those to the metacarpals, nasals, and proximal phalanges are relatively minor injuries that would minimally impede an individual's ability to move and work. Contemporary surgeons referred to fractured fingers as trivial cases (Bristowe and Holmes, 1864). Lay first-aid was often adequate; Roy Porter asserts that "experienced and careful lay people could handle most accidents, even serious-sounding conditions such as fractures" (1997, p. 96). William Buchan, in his landmark publication *Domestic Medicine*, in reference to fractures, notes that

> there is in most country villages some person who pretends to the art of reducing fractures. Though in general such persons are very ignorant, yet some of them are very successful; which evidently proves, that a small degree of learning, with a sufficient share of common sense and a mechanical head, will enable a man to be useful in this way
>
> *(1769, p. 722).*

Buchan does, however, caution that "we would however advise people never to trust such operators, when an expert and skillful surgeon can be had; but when that is impracticable, they must be employed" (1769, p. 722). In cases where a fracture was deemed minor, or the hospital admissions procedure was too laborious, or a governor's recommendation was unprocurable, or the fees charged by the local physician were too expensive, "every man is in some measure a surgeon whether he will or not" (Buchan, 1769, p. 695). It must be considered that "medicine was a business as well as a vocation" (Digby, 1994, p. 19) and the medical marketplace served individuals who could afford to pay for their care. The working poor often could not afford the services of a physician and therefore relied upon lay medical knowledge or the voluntary hospitals of London.

The patterns displayed in Figs. 4.6 and 4.7 suggest that male and female risk factors for leg fractures may be age-related. The lack of fracture location data limits the comparability of these data with many clinical and epidemiological studies. Clinically, the relationship between increasing age and increasing incidence of hip fractures has been documented (Poole et al., 2010) with females sustaining hip fractures at an average age of 77 and males at an average age of 72 (Baumgaertner and Higgins, 2002). Age-related bone loss and increased bone fragility may be possible complicating factors in the hospital admissions sample, but this supposition remains necessarily speculative. The relatively small sample group of individuals in the older adult age groups (61–90 years; males n = 105/1910; females n = 54/1250) may indicate that fewer older adult individuals were suffering fractures in the past, but it is more likely that older individuals may not have sought hospital care for fractures due to decreased mobility and senescence. Alternatively, age bias may have been present in the original admissions. Various contemporary sources note that individuals accepted into the general hospitals should be "deserving" or "worthy objects of charity" (Woodward, 1974, p. 40), since the hospitals were serving to "[recover] future wealth potentially lost to the nation" (Lawrence, 1996, p. 45). The potential of individuals in these older age groups to contribute meaningfully to the economy was likely viewed as limited.

The intangible notion of human choice is represented in the results of this case study. Minor injuries to the fingers and toes, as well as myriad rib fractures, outrank major femoral fractures in the skeletal remains; essentially the opposite result is found in the hospital admissions registers. These results reveal personal choices made in the past in reference to an individual's health; the results suggest that males and females were seeking hospital admission for similar reasons. In some cases individuals did not make their own choice to go to hospital, perhaps because they were injured in a public place, particularly in the case of accidents involving vehicles, and were rushed to a hospital by friends or bystanders. These victims were often unconscious or "found quite insensible," such as John West, admitted to St. George's, having been "thrown from off a stage coach and pitched upon his head" (Royal College of Surgeons, 1805–1851, MS0470 62, p. 31).

In most cases, however, individuals dealt with the situation described by Wilde (1810), the actor and poet, who, upon arriving at the Devon and Exeter hospital, found "himself amongst a crowd/Of wretched candidates to gain admission;/Each recommended by some kind subscriber" (p. 6). Wilde was nearly rejected due to his lack of governor or subscriber's recommendation, "alas! [he] had fail'd through lack of forms / And now, his long, and agonizing journey / Had all abortive prov'd" (1810, p. 6). Thankfully, Wilde managed to connect with "a friend—and one more true, / Or swifter to obey the call of pity, / Ne'er trod the earth...So should the name of PEAR, the parish clerk, / Descend to ages" (1810, p. 5); this individual secured Wilde the appropriate recommendation paperwork.

4.6 CONCLUSIONS

This research reveals distinct differences between the lives of working poor males and females who lived and died in London during the 18th and early 19th centuries. The skeletal results demonstrate that males suffered more fractures than females overall and in different areas of the body, suggesting that males and females were at differential risk for various types of fracture. Overall, leg fractures appear in abundance in the admission records, while rib fractures are the most numerous in the skeletal dataset. Evidence of decision-making regarding health care in the past is accessible through this research. The results demonstrate that males and females were seeking hospital admission for fractures to similar anatomical groups (ie, leg, arm, rib/ribs), despite the fact that fracture frequencies differ significantly between males and females in both the skeletal and admission records datasets and the age at which these fractures occurred differs between the sexes.

The decision to seek hospital admission depended upon a complex nexus of factors including: securing transport to the hospital's location, weighing the hospital's reputation for curing patients, acquiring a governor's guarantee, weighing of the effect of possible wages lost during convalescence, and determining whether or not an alternative practitioner could effectively treat the fracture at home. This bioarch-aeological study lends credence to historians' examinations of attitudes concerning 18th-century hospital care (eg, Porter, 1997) and provides evidence to further studies of alternative medicine. Identifying which fractures were not commonly recorded in the hospital admission records provides a picture of which injuries were most commonly being treated in the home or with the assistance of other members of the medical marketplace. These disparate lines of data speak in concert to provide insight into the vibrant and vital world of 18th-century health care, its stakeholders, and their choices.

ACKNOWLEDGMENTS

Thank you to Dr. Rebecca Redfern and Jelena Bekvalac of the Museum of London Centre for Human Bioarchaeology for allowing access to the RLP05 skeletal collection and database. Jonathan Evans and Richard Meunier of the Royal London Hospital Museum and Archives provided access to the hospital admission books. Thank you to Drs. Ann Herring and Megan Brickley for their insightful comments, which greatly improved the quality of this manuscript. Thank you also to Drs. Becky Redfern and Anne Grauer, whose critiques were exceptionally helpful in improving the clarity of this paper.

REFERENCES

Arrizabalaga, J., 2002. Problematizing retrospective diagnosis in the history of disease. Asclepio 54, 51–70.

Baumgaertner, M.R., Higgins, T.F., 2002. Femoral neck fractures. In: Bucholz, R.W., Heckman, J.D., Rockwood, C.A., Green, D.P. (Eds.), Rockwood and Green's Fractures in Adults. Lippincott Williams & Wilkins, Philadelphia, PA, p. 1579.

Brickley, M., 2006. Rib fractures in the archaeological record: a useful source of sociocultural information? Int. J. Osteoarchaeol. 16, 61–75.

Bristowe, J.S., Holmes, T., 1864. Report on the hospitals of the United Kingdom. Sixth Report of the Medical Officer of the Privy Council, 1863. George E. Eyre and William Spottiswoode, for her Majesty's Stationery Office, London.

Brodie, B., 1805–1807. Surgical Cases and Commentaries, vol. 1. Royal College of Surgeons of England Archives, MS0470 38.

Brooks, S.T., Suchey, J.M., 1990. Skeletal age determination based on the os pubis: a comparison of the Acsádi-Nemeskéri and Suchey-Brooks methods. Hum. Evolut. 5, 227–238.

Brothwell, D.R., 1981. Digging Up Bones, third ed. British Museum (Natural History), London.

Buchan, J., 1769. Domestic Medicine: or, a Treatise on the Prevention and Cure of Diseases by Regiment and Simple Medicines. Balfour, Auld & Smellie, Edinburgh.

Buhr, A.J., Cooke, A.M., 1959. Fracture patterns. Lancet531−536, March 14, 1959.

Buikstra, J.E., Ubelaker, D.H. (Eds.), 1994. Standards for data collection from human skeletal remains. Arkansas Archaeological Survey Research Series No. 44, Arkansas.

Carruthers, G.B., Carruthers, L.A., 2005. A History of Britain's Hospitals. Book Guild Publishing, Sussex.

Chamberlain, A., 2012. Morbid osteology: evidence for autopsies, dissection and surgical training from the Newcastle Infirmary Burial Ground (1753−1845). In: Mitchell, P. (Ed.), Anatomical Dissection in Enlightenment England and Beyond. Ashgate, Farnham, pp. 11−22.

Chaplin, S., 2012. Dissection and display in eighteenth-century London. In: Mitchell, P. (Ed.), Anatomical Dissection in Enlightenment England and Beyond. Ashgate, Farnham, pp. 95−114.

Chodorow, S., 2006. To represent us truly: the job and context of preserving the cultural record. Libr. Cult. Rec. 41, 372−380.

Clark-Kennedy, A.E., 1962. The London: A Study in the Voluntary Hospital System, vol. 1. Pitman Medical Publishing Co. Ltd., London, pp. 1740−1840.

Court-Brown, C.M., Caesar, B., 2006. Epidemiology of adult fractures: a review. Injury 37, 691−697.

Cullen, W., 1792. Synopsis and Nosology, Being an Arrangement of Diseases. Nathaniel Patten, Hartford.

Cunningham, A., 2002. Identifying disease in the past: cutting the Gordian knot. Asclepio 54, 13−34.

Dainton, C., 1961. The Story of England's Hospitals. Charles C. Thomas, Springfield.

Digby, A., 1994. Making a Medical Living: Doctors and Patients in the English Market for Medicine, 1720−1911. Cambridge University Press, Cambridge, MA.

Donaldson, L.J., Cook, A., Thomson, R.G., 1990. Incidence of fractures in a geographically defined population. J. Epidemiol. Commun. Health 44, 241−245.

Drake, M. (Ed.), 1982. Population Studies from Parish Registers. G. C. Brittain & Sons Ltd., Derby.

Dyson, R., 2014. How did the poor cope with illness: perspectives from early nineteenth-century Oxford. Fam. Commun. Hist. 17, 86−100.

Fowler, L., Powers, N., 2012a. Doctors, Dissection and Resurrection Men: Excavations in the 19th-century Burial Ground of the London Hospital, 2006. Museum of London Archaeology, London, Monograph 62.

Fowler, L., Powers, N., 2012b. Patients, anatomists and resurrection men: archaeological evidence for anatomy teaching at the London hospital in the early nineteenth century. In: Mitchell, P. (Ed.), Anatomical Dissection in Enlightenment England and Beyond. Ashgate, Farnham, pp. 77−94.

Ginzburg, C., 1989. Clues, Myths, and the Historical Method (T.J. Tedeschi, A.C. Tedeschi, Trans.). The Johns Hopkins University Press, Baltimore, MD.

Glencross, B.A., 2011. Skeletal injury across the life course: towards understanding social agency. In: Agarwal, S.C., Glencross, B. (Eds.), Social Bioarchaeology. Wiley-Blackwell, London, pp. 390−409.

Glencross, B., Sawchuk, L., 2003. The person-years construct: ageing and the prevalence of health related phenomena from skeletal samples. Int. J. Osteoarchaeol. 13, 369−374.

Grauer, A.L., 1995. Preface. In: Grauer, A.L. (Ed.), Bodies of Evidence: Reconstructing History through Skeletal Analysis. Wiley-Liss, New York, NY, pp. ix−x.

Hays, J.N., 2007. Historians and epidemics: simple questions, complex answers. In: Little, L.K. (Ed.), Plague and the End of Antiquity: The Pandemic of 541−750. Cambridge University Press, Cambridge, MA, pp. 33−56.

Hoppa, R.D., Vaupel, J.W. (Eds.), 2002. Paleodemography: Age Distributions From Skeletal Samples. Cambridge University Press, Cambridge, MA.

Howard, J., 1791. An Account of the Principal Lazarettos in Europe, second ed. London, Printed for J. Johnson, C. Dilly, and T. Cadell.

Howell, N., 1986. Demographic anthropology. Annu. Rev. Anthropol. 15, 219–306.

Isçan, M., Loth, S., 1986a. Determination of age from the sternal rib in white males: a test of the phase method. J. Forensic Sci. 31, 122–132.

Isçan, M., Loth, S., 1986b. Determination of age from the sternal rib in white females: a test of the phase method. J. Forensic Sci. 31, 990–999.

Johansen, A., Evans, R.J., Stone, M.D., Richmond, P.W., Lo, S.V., Woodhouse, K.W., 1997. Fracture incidence in England and Wales: a study based on the population of Cardiff. Injury 28, 655–660.

Jurmain, R., 1999. Stories From the Skeleton, Behavioural Reconstruction in Human Osteology. Taylor & Francis, London.

Kara, M., Dikmen, E., Erdal, H.H., Simsir, I., Kara, S.A., 2003. Disclosure of unnoticed rib fractures with use of ultrasonography in minor blunt chest trauma. Eur. J. Cardio-Thorac. 24, 608–613.

King, L.S., 1958. The Medical World of the Eighteenth Century. Robert E. Krieger Publishing, Chicago, IL.

King's College London, 1725-1726. Surgical student's notebook, St. Thomas' Hospital. GB 0100 TH/PP44.

Koval, K.J., Cooley, M., 2006. Experience in the United States. In: Bucholz, R.W., Heckman, J.D., Court-Brown, C.M. (Eds.), Rockwood and Green's Fractures in Adults, sixth ed. Lippincott Williams & Wilkins, Philadelphia, PA, pp. 113–143.

Kramaker, M.K., Anthony, M., 2003. Acute pain management of patients with multiple fractured ribs. J. Trauma 53, 615–625.

Lane, J., 2001. A Social History of Medicine: Health, Healing and Disease in England, 1750–1950. Routledge, London and New York.

Langford, P., 1989. A Polite and Commercial People. England 1727–1783. Clarendon Press, Oxford.

Lawrence, S.C., 1996. Charitable Knowledge: Hospital Pupils and Practitioners in Eighteenth-Century London. Cambridge University Press, Cambridge, MA.

Levene, A., 2006. General introduction. In: King, S., Nutt, T., Tomkins, A. (Eds.), Narratives of the Poor in Eighteenth-Century Britain, vol. 1. Pickering & Chatto, London, pp. vii–xix.

Lovejoy, C.O., Meindl, R.S., Pryzbeck, T.R., Mensforth, R.P., 1985. Chronological metamorphosis of the auricular surface of the ilium: a new method for the determination of age at death. Am. J. Phys. Anthropol. 68, 47–56.

Metcalfe, N.H., 2007. A description of the methods used to obtain information on ancient disease and medicine and of how the evidence has survived. Postgrad. Med. J. 83, 655–658.

Mitchell, P.D., 2011. Retrospective diagnosis and the use of historical texts for investigating disease in the past. Int. J. Palaeopath. 1, 81–88.

Mitchell, P.D., 2012. Integrating historical sources with paleopathology. In: Grauer, A.L. (Ed.), A Companion to Paleopathology. Wiley-Blackwell, Chichester, pp. 310–323.

Mitchell, P.D., Chauhan, V., 2012. Understanding the contents of the Westminster Hospital pathology museum in the 1800s. In: Mitchell, P. (Ed.), Anatomical Dissection in Enlightenment England and Beyond: Autopsy, Pathology and Display. Ashgate, Farnham, pp. 140–154.

Mitchell, P.D., Boston, C., Chamberlain, A.T., Chaplin, S., Chauhan, V., Evans, J., et al., 2011. The study of anatomy in England from 1700 to the early 20th century. J. Anat. 219, 91–99.

Newell, C., 1988. Methods and Models in Demography. The Guilford Press, New York, NY.

A descriptive catalogue of the anatomical museum of St. Bartholomew's Hospital. In: Paget, J. Containing the descriptions of the specimens illustrative of pathological anatomy, vol. 1. John Churchill, London.

Petersen, W., 1975. A demographer's view of prehistoric demography. Curr. Anthropol. 16, 227–245.

Poole, K.E., Mayhew, P.M., Rose, C.M., Brown, J.K., Bearcroft, P.J., Loveridge, N., et al., 2010. Changing structure of the femoral neck across the adult lifespan. J. Bone Miner. Res. 25, 482–491.

Porter, R., 1997. Accidents in the eighteenth century. In: Cooter, R., Luckin, B. (Eds.), Accidents in History: Injuries, Fatalities and Social Relations. Rodopi, Amsterdam, pp. 90–106.

Powers, N. (Ed.), 2012. Human Osteology Method Statement. Museum of London, London.

Risse, G.B., 1986. Hospital Life in Enlightenment Scotland: Care and Teaching at the Royal Infirmary of Edinburgh. Cambridge University Press, Cambridge, MA.

Rivett, G., 1986. The Development of the London Hospital System, 1823–1982. Oxford University Press, Oxford.

Roberts, C.A., Cox, M., 2003. Health & Disease in Britain: From Prehistory to the Present Day. Sutton, Stroud.

Rosenberg, C.E., Golden, J. (Eds.), 1992. Framing Disease: Studies in Cultural History. Rutgers University Press, New Brunswick, NJ.

Royal College of Surgeons, 1805. Case Histories for the Years 1805–1851. St. George's Hospital, London, MS0470.

Royal Infirmary of Edinburgh, 1770. Minute Book, MSS Collection, Medical Archives, University of Edinburgh, vol. 4, meeting of August 6, 1770.

Sahlin, Y., 1990. Occurrence of fractures in a defined population: a 1-year study. Injury 21, 158–160.

Siegel, J.S., Swanson, D.A., 2004. The Methods and Materials of Demography. Elsevier Academic Press Inc., London.

Singer, B.R., McLauchlan, G.J., Robinson, C.M., Christie, J., 1998. Epidemiology of fractures in 15 000 adults. J. Bone Joint. Surg. Br. 80-B, 243–248.

Tekinbas, C., Eroglu, A., Kurkcuoglu, I.C., Turkyilmaz, A., Yekeler, E., Yavuz, C., 2003. Chest trauma analysis of 529 cases. Ulus. Travma Acil. Cer. 9, 275–280.

Turkel, W.J., 2006. Every place is an archive: environmental history and the interpretation of physical evidence. Rethink. Hist 10, 259–276.

United Nations, 1955. Methods of appraisal of quality of basic data for population estimates, Manual II. United Nations Population Studies, No. 23, New York.

van Staa, T.P., Dennison, E.M., Leufkens, H.G.M., Cooper, C., 2001. Epidemiology of fractures in England and Wales. Bone 29, 517–522.

Waldron, T., 1991. Rates for the job. Measures of disease frequency in palaeopathology. Int. J. Osteoarch. 1, 17–25.

Warden, S.J., Gutschlag, F.R., Wajswelner, H., Crossley, K.M., 2002. Aetiology of rib stress fractures in rower. Sports Med. 32, 819–836.

Wilde, J., 1810. The Hospital, A Poem in Three Books, Written in the Devon & Exeter Hospital, 1809. Stevenson, Matchett, and Stevenson, Norwich.

Winks, R.W. (Ed.), 1969. The Historian as Detective: Essays on Evidence. Harper & Row, New York, NY.

Woodward, J., 1974. To Do the Sick No Harm. A Study of the British Voluntary Hospital System to 1875. Routledge & Kegan Paul, London.

CHAPTER 5

Reading Between the Lines: Disparate Data and Castration Studies

K. Reusch

School of Archaeology, University of Oxford, Oxford, United Kingdom

5.1 INTRODUCTION

Castration[1] has been intertwined with human history throughout Afro-Eurasia for millennia. Possibly beginning with the Secondary Products Revolution (SPR) (Chalcolithic to Bronze Age, roughly 6200–4500 BCE) (Greenfield, 2010; Orton, 2014; Sherratt, 1983; Taylor, 2002) in the Fertile Crescent (Scholz, 2001; Tougher, 2002, 2008), castration spread through ancient empires, including the Assyrian, Roman, Chinese, Byzantine, Islamic, and Ottoman (Doran, 2010; El-Cheikh, 2005; Marmon, 1995; Matthews, 1994; Mitamura, 1970; Tougher, 2002, 2008, 2013), and religions, including the cult of the *Magna Mater*/Cybele, Bahuchara Mata, and various Christian sects, from ancient times, through the *castrati*[2] singers, to the USSR in the 1950s CE (Barbier, 1998; Engelstein, 1999; Lane, 1978; Mukherjee, 1980; Nanda, 1999; Scholz, 2001; Vermaseren, 1977), and even to the modern day with the use of chemical castration for criminals and prostate cancer patients (Aucoin and Wassersug, 2006; Brett

---

[1]Castration is here defined as the removal of either the testicles or the testicles and the penis. This was referred to in Reusch (2013b) as partial and complete castration, respectively, however, the technical terms are actually castration and castration with penectomy. Both forms have been practiced throughout human history, as far as can be discerned, with removal of the testicles only most popular in Europe and portions of the Fertile Crescent and removal of both testicles and penis most popular in Africa, portions of the Fertile Crescent, and Asia. In animals, only the testicles are removed, to the author's knowledge.

[2]Historically, there have been a number of terms used to refer to castrated individuals. The two most popular terms have been *castrati* and *eunuch*. Both terms have specific cultural and historical meanings (*castrati* is used to refer specifically to the European singers employed by opera and church choirs in the Early Modern period and *eunuch* comes from a Greek term meaning "guardian of the bedchamber" and refers to castrated servants' employment in the domestic sphere of households), and have therefore been used only in those appropriate settings within this paper. All other references to castrated persons will use the term castrate.

Beyond the Bones. DOI: http://dx.doi.org/10.1016/B978-0-12-804601-2.00005-3

et al., 2007). Several fields have contributed to the study of castration throughout time, including history, medicine, archaeology, paleopathology, zooarchaeology, gender studies, and sexuality studies (Beard, 2012; Davis, 2000; Dreger, 1998; Eng et al., 2010; Fausto-Sterling, 2000; Ringrose, 2003; Scholz, 2001; Tougher, 2008; Wilson and Roehrborn, 1999). Castration's development, early history, and physical and social effects are, however, not well understood, especially within the medico-anthropological literature.

Castrates form a group of historically visible, often extremely powerful, intersex individuals. Through their connection to rulers and religion, castrates were often positioned to affect the policies of many hierarchical organizations with secular and religious political control. They are often upbraided in historical documents *because* of their ability to adversely affect rulers and kingdoms (Scholz, 2001; Tougher, 2008; Tsai, 1996). They also formed a highly visible third gender category in many societies (Herdt, 1994; Ringrose, 1994), which may have affected wider societal views of sex and gender norms. Despite their great influence on human history, very little is actually known about castrates as individuals or as a group. Castrates are an artificially constructed intersex category, but naturally intersex individuals have existed throughout recorded human history (Dreger, 1998; Leick, 2003; Reis, 2005). As only one intersex skeleton has ever been identified archaeologically (Ghosh, 2015), the ability to better recognize intersex individuals would allow the history of these conditions to be traced through time, adding depth to our current clinical understanding.

This work stems from a doctoral project that was originally undertaken to determine the effects of prepubertal castration on the development of the male skeleton, which changed to a multifold, interdisciplinary examination of the effects of castration in order to more clearly delineate skeletal change and aid castrate identification. This project required a careful literature review to find casual anecdotes and throwaway references, as well as gaining access to obscure papers and the private notes of previous castration scholars. Gender, sex, sexuality, and identity literature covering both past and modern societies was consulted in order to formulate ideas of how castrates may have perceived themselves both as a group and within their wider societies. Modern medical and endocrinological literature was consulted in order to understand the possible physical effects of castration. Given the lack of human remains available for study, it was necessary to consult zooarchaeological and veterinary studies of castration to determine which changes were common across mammalian species and therefore likely due to the castration. The project sought to bring these disparate strands of data together to create a comprehensive and coherent narrative of social and skeletal change that could be used to identify castrate skeletons within archaeological collections in the future.

5.2 ESTABLISHING THE ORIGIN, SPREAD, AND HISTORICAL PRESENCE OF CASTRATION

Castration and castrates have been woven through human historical documents for millennia. Usually associated with kings, elites, and power, human castrates appear to have thrived once hierarchical power structures became common (most likely by the 4th millennium BCE) (Taylor, 2002). They tend to fall into two major categories, castrates associated with rulers and castrates associated with religions, though some blending between the categories could exist, depending on the power structures inherent in a society (Reusch, 2013a). However, in some societies, such as the Byzantine Empire, castrates could be found in all social strata, from court officials to prostitutes (Ringrose, 2003; Tougher, 2008).

Based on available zooarchaeological information, animal castration seems to have begun around the SPR (Greenfield, 2010; Sherratt, 1983), during which castration is thought to have been developed as a method of retaining male animals past the 2-year growth period normal for meat and milk (primary products) production. The prolonged life of the castrated animals gave the benefit of secondary products such as wool and draught labor, while castration protected already well-established breeding programs. Getting secure dates for the beginning of animal castration is difficult, due to the limitations of detecting castrated animals within the archaeological record (Davis, 2000).

The first possible references to human castration come from Uruk (~4000 BCE), in the myths of the cult of the goddess Ishtar/Inanna, especially "The Descent of Inanna"[3] (Taylor, 2002). The next potential indications come from other Mesopotamian cultures such as Sumer, Ur, the Akkadian Empire, and the Assyrian Empire ($\sim$3rd Millenium−1st Millenium BCE) (Asher-Greve, 1997; Dalley, 2002; Siddall, 2007; Tadmor, 1983), in visual art and textual references to the *ša reši*, or man with two heads, which has controversially been taken to mean eunuch (Briant, 2002; Tougher, 2008). From this, it seems that either sometime between the SPR and the formation of the hierarchical, religious civilizations of Mesopotamia, or in concert with the development of animal castration during the SPR, the castration of animals was carried over into humans. This was possibly a side effect of war and slavery, or the formation of social hierarchies (Coughlan, 2012; Taylor, 2002). It is probable that the formation of the stratified, hierarchical societies made possible by agriculture led to the conceptualization of lower status people or prisoners of war as comparable to animals, making their castration a matter of population control (Taylor, 2002). Alternately, it is possible that the use of intersex individuals within daily life, temple rituals, and court functions (Leick, 2003) became normalized during this period, resulting in the production of artificially intersexed people through human castration when "natural supply" (natural-born intersex individuals) was not enough to meet demand.

Castration soon spread throughout the Fertile Crescent and surrounding areas. The Mesopotamian sources are followed by possible references in Egyptian documents (from the 19th Dynasty, c.1300 BCE) (Kadish, 1969) and descriptions in Persian and Greek documents (Llewellyn-Jones, 2002; Patterson, 1982; Tougher, 2008). Chinese oracle bones use the characters for eunuch from at least 1300 BCE (Jay, 1993; Tsai, 1996). Once the Romans brought the cult of Cybele, also known as the *Magna Mater*, to Rome in 204 BCE, castration became fairly commonplace in the Mediterranean basin (especially the eastern portion) through the spread of castrated *galli* priests and household servants (Beard, 2012; Tougher, 2013; Vermaseren, 1977). By the time the capital of the Roman Empire moved to Constantinople (CE 323), castrates were

---

[3]While these myths largely come from Protoliterate Period (2900−2750 BCE) cuneiform tablets found in the Ishtar temple complex in Uruk, it is generally agreed by scholars that these myths are older than the surviving written forms, that castrates were associated with the cult at an early period, and that the cult originated in Uruk probably in the early Uruk period (4500−3750 BCE) (Bi and Xiao, 2009; Taylor, 2002).

in charge of the emperor's household and held several positions within government (Ringrose, 2003; Scholz, 2001; Tougher, 2008). When the Ottomans conquered Constantinople in CE 1453, castrates continued to serve at court, but in slightly modified roles (Scholz, 2001; Segal, 2001). Islamic countries had utilized castrates heavily within military, political, and administrative roles from the Abbasid dynasty (CE 750−1258). They spread their use at royal courts across Afro-Eurasia from India and Central Asia to the Iberian Peninsula and North and Central Africa (Marmon, 1995; Segal, 2001; Ware, 2011), but the Turkish court was one of the largest Islamic consumers of castrates (Fig. 5.1).

Meanwhile in China, eunuchs expanded into several aspects of court life, including serving in the government by the Zhou Dynasty (1045−256 BCE) (Kutcher, 2010). After Qin unification (221 BCE), eunuchs worked as gatekeepers, servants, and messengers in the palace, slowly gaining full control of the domestic affairs of the imperial palace over millennia (Jay, 1993; Scholz, 2001). Under the influence

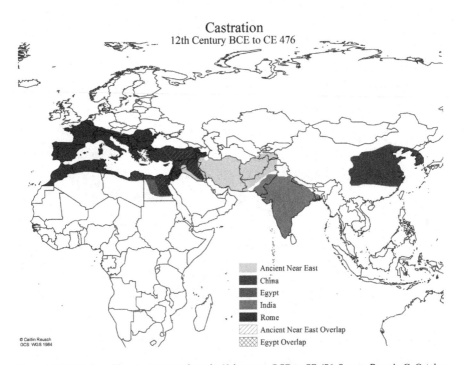

Figure 5.1 Distribution of human castration from the 12th century BCE to CE 476. Source: Reusch, C. October 1, 2015. Early Castration: 12th Century BCE to 476 CE [map], first ed. 1:69,510,943; Base world map citation: Erle, S. July 30, 2008. *TM_WORLD_BORDERS-0.1* [GIS shapefile], third ed. <http://www.mappinghacks. com/data/ > (accessed 01.10.15).

of the Ming Dynasty (CE 1368–1644), castration spread to the royal courts of Korea and Vietnam, which also sent eunuchs as tribute to the Chinese capital during both the Ming and the Qing (CE 1644–1912) Dynasties (Jay, 1993; Mitamura, 1970).

In India, historic castration is more difficult to follow. Castration is mentioned in Vedic sacred texts (1500–1000 BCE) (Bullough, 2002), and eunuchs served in Mughal courts (CE 1526–1857) (Scholz, 2001), but the castrates for which India is most famous are the *hijras*. Devotees of Bahuchara Mata, they dress as women and sing, dance, and offer blessings at weddings and the birth of sons (Mukherjee, 1980; Nanda, 1999; Preston, 1987). They have existed from before the British conquest of India (CE 1817–18) to the modern day, though not all modern *hijras* are castrated (Preston, 1987; Scholz, 2001) (Fig. 5.2).

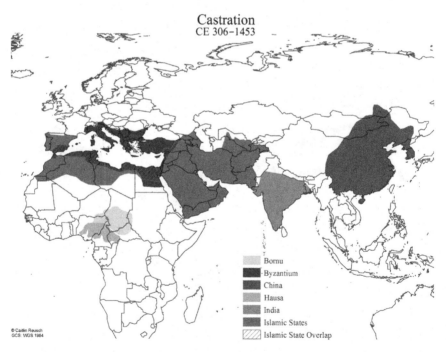

Castration
CE 306–1453

Bornu
Byzantium
China
Hausa
India
Islamic States
Islamic State Overlap

© Caitlin Reusch
GCS: WGS 1984

Figure 5.2 Distribution of human castration from CE 306 to 1453. Source: Reusch, C., October 1, 2015. Middle Castration: 306 to 1453 CE [map], first ed. 1:69,510,943; Base world map citation: Erle, S., July 30, 2008. *TM_WORLD_BORDERS-0.1* [GIS shapefile], third ed. <http://www.mappinghacks.com/data/> (accessed 01.10.15).

The castrates most familiar to Western audiences are the *castrati* singers of the Baroque and later periods in Europe (16th–20th centuries CE). There is some confusion as to when exactly the Papal chapel first admitted castrated singers (Gerbino, 2004), but in CE 1589, Pope Sixtus V issued a bull which officially included four individuals explicitly described as castrates in the choir, and in CE 1594, Pope Clement VIII allowed Italian *castrati* to join the choir (Gerbino, 2004; Jenkins, 1998; Milner, 1973). By CE 1640, *castrati* were found in church choirs across Italy, and many had become operatic stars (Jenkins, 1998; Rosselli, 1988). Although the taste for *castrati* in opera and wider church choirs faded over time, they were still employed in the papal choir until Pope Leo XIII prohibited their creation and addition to the choir in CE 1878 (Bullough, 2002). Alessandro Moreschi, the last *castrati*, died in CE 1922 (Scholz, 2001).

Christianity was involved with castration from its earliest days, as several church fathers had self-castrated as a sign of devotion and chastity (Scholz, 2001). The major motivation for *castrati* as singers was a perceived prohibition of women singing in church choirs (Barbier, 1998; Scholz, 2001). The Christian sect associated with castration that has received the most attention and concern from authorities is the Skoptsy. Springing from an offshoot of Russian Orthodox Christianity around CE 1700, this sect practiced self-castration and breast mutilation in an effort to remove "impure" signifiers of sex within humans (Engelstein, 1999; Tandler and Grosz, 1910). The Romanov (CE 1613–1917) and succeeding Bolshevik (CE 1917–22) and Soviet (CE 1922–91) governments tried to eradicate the sect, which caused many members to flee to Romania, where they set up several successful settlements (Pittard, 1934; Wilson and Roehrborn, 1999). It is thought that the sect died out in the 1950s CE (Engelstein, 1999) (Fig. 5.3).

From the study of the historical spread of castration, it is possible to determine where best to target searches for castrated remains, as well as to show archaeologists and paleopathologists where they need to be mindful of finding castrate skeletons within larger skeletal populations. This research also highlights the great number of historically important cultures that employed castrates, often in close proximity to rulers whose thinking they could influence. This often led to jealousy and competition with intact male courtiers and bureaucrats, who viewed castrates as part-males, feminine in nature, or semihuman

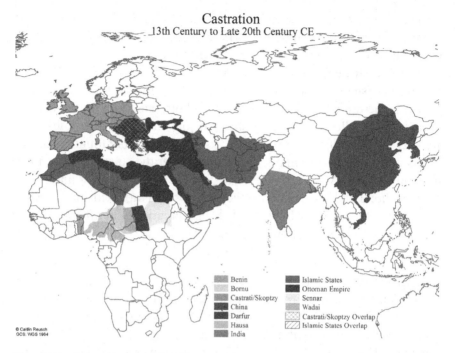

Figure 5.3 Distribution of human castration from the 13th-late 20th centuries CE. Source: Reusch, C. October 1, 2015. Late Castration: 13th Century to Late 20th Century CE [map], first ed. 1:69,510,943; Base world map citation: Erle, S. July 30, 2008. *TM_WORLD_BORDERS-0.1* [GIS shapefile], third ed. <http://www.mappin-ghacks.com/data/> (accessed 01.10.15).

monsters (Magie, 1924; Patterson, 1982; Scholz, 2001; Tougher, 1997). As these individuals were the ones most often writing about castrates, both historical and modern perceptions of castrates have been colored, affecting how and by whom they have been studied.

5.3 ESTABLISHING THE PHYSICAL EFFECTS OF CASTRATION

5.3.1 Historical Accounts of the Effects of Castration

Several historical authors have addressed the effects of castration on both male physiology and psychology. Sometimes these accounts were used to denigrate castrates themselves or teach moral lessons about the evils of castration and castrates. Herodotus described the revenge one of Xerxes' eunuchs took upon his castrator (Hornblower, 2003). Aristotle gave the first real account of the effects of prepubertal castration in animals and humans, noting their inability to procreate or develop secondary sexual characteristics, seemingly making castrates female (Aristotle, 1984 (8(9).50)). Galen agreed with Aristotle's contention that castrates were essentially men made into women (Ringrose, 1999), and this view of castrates continued into the present day, affecting the labeling of figures in ancient art, especially from the Fertile Crescent and Egypt, as castrates if they appear male but with long limbs, a small head, breast development, round hips, a lack of a beard, and slight to morbid obesity (Kadish, 1969; Ringrose, 1999).

Late Ottoman eunuchs were described as thin, but with increasing fat as they aged, having wrinkled faces, jutting teeth, stunted chins, and long, flabby limbs and short torsos (von Bayern, 1923). The Chinese thought of castrates as never having beards or body hair but also avoiding male balding, as having high-pitched voices, disproportionately long limbs, and fat over the hips, buttocks, and breasts, as well as looking attractive in their youth, gaining weight in their middle age, and looking feminine when they aged (Jay, 1993). *Castrati* were called boyish and effeminate, possessing female speaking voices, disproportionate limbs, small heads and shoulders, plentiful head hair, beardless faces, wrinkles late in life, breasts, a tendency to obesity, large, rounded pelves, and "barrel" chests, likely due to their intensive vocal training (Freitas, 2003; Jenkins, 1998, 2001; Krimmer, 2005; Potter, 2007). *Hijras* have been described as feminine, possessing high-pitched voices, slender, delicate limbs, fat on the buttocks and legs, and a disproportionate upper to lower body ratio (Mukherjee, 1980).

Studies of castrates carried out in the late 19th and early 20th centuries CE began to refine the understanding of the skeletal effects of castration. These studies, carried out to understand the processes of castration and its relation to the dawning field of endocrinology, took one of two forms: osteometric (skeletal) or anthropometric (living individuals). The osteometric studies were Lortet's study of a castrate of Shilluk (Nilotic) origin now held in Lyon, France (Lortet, 1896), the examination of Nekht-Ankh, a 12th Dynasty (1991–1783 BCE) aristocratic mummy excavated in Rifeh, Egypt (Murray, 1910), and Tandler and Grosz's autopsy of a Zanzibarian castrate who died in the Rudolfsspitale in Vienna, Austria (Tandler and Grosz, 1909). These studies stated that castrate skeletons were often gracile and fine boned, with few strongly defined muscle insertion points, as well as possessing extremely long axial skeletons, often with still open epiphyses. The skulls and pelves were described as small and childlike, with disproportionally longer lower limbs than torsos.

The anthropometric studies included: Tandler and Grosz's examination of five Skoptsy men in Bucharest (Tandler and Grosz, 1910); followed by Koch's study of 13 Skoptsy men in Romania during World War I (Koch, 1921); then Wagenseil's descriptions of 11 Ottoman palace eunuchs of sub-Saharan African origin (Wagenseil, 1927) and 31 Chinese palace eunuchs (Wagenseil, 1933); and finally Pittard's examination of 30 Skoptsy men in Romania before World War I (Pittard, 1934). Common results of these studies were extreme length in the axial skeleton, disproportionate limb-to-torso length and *genu valgum* (knock knees), tall and narrow faces, enlarged pelves, kyphosis of the spine, tall and thin or fat body types, and the knowledge that earlier castration resulted in more extreme effects (Koch, 1921; Pittard, 1934; Tandler and Grosz, 1910; Wagenseil, 1927, 1933). The data contained within these reports provide an invaluable resource for castrate measurements, something that can no longer be easily obtained, as castrates no longer exist in large numbers and it is unethical to refuse treatment to intersex individuals out of scientific curiosity. These data were used in comparison with the modern paleopathologically obtained data in order to more fully describe the changes to the castrate skeleton, as well as for statistical analyses.

5.3.2 Modern Clinical and Anthropological Accounts of the Effects of Castration

Medicine, endocrinology, and animal studies can indicate what skeletal effects to expect from prepubertal castration. Animals castrated before puberty experience an elongation of the limbs similar to humans (Armitage and Clutton-Brock, 1976; Dahinten and Pucciarelli, 1986; Davis, 2000). Endocrinology shows that the reason for the skeletal changes stems from the loss of the testes, the major producer of androgens (male sex hormones) (Hiort, 2002; Hiort et al., 2007; Vanderschueren et al., 1998; Winters and Clark, 2003). Without androgens, skeletal masculinization cannot occur and epiphyseal fusion is delayed, because some androgens are turned into estrogens (female sex hormones), which halt bone growth (Kenny and Raisz, 2003; Vanderschueren et al., 1998). Without the main source of hormonal differentiation, male skeletons default to a more female state, resulting in intersex skeletons. This is often seen in individuals with congenital intersex conditions such as anorchia (Hegarty et al., 2007; Vinci et al., 2004), primary hypogonadism (Jay, 1993; Plymate, 2003), congenital hypogonadotropic eunuchoidism, testicular trauma, and androgen or

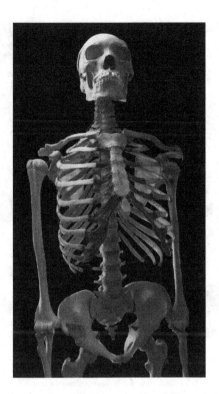

Figure 5.4 Axial skeleton of the Lyon castrate, displaying the open epiphyses, elongated humeri, expanded ribs, and unusual morphology of the skull and pelvic girdle. Source: Photo by author.

estrogen insensitivity syndromes (Plymate, 2003; Quigley et al., 1995; Winters and Clark, 2003). Most of these individuals are treated with hormones once their condition is discovered, making it difficult to use their measurements in comparison with archaeological castrates (Plymate, 2003; Quigley et al., 1995) (Fig. 5.4).

While few human castrate skeletons are readily available for examination, there have been skeletons discussed in the literature. Eng and colleagues (2010) described the skeletons of two Ming Dynasty eunuchs recovered during the excavation of a cemetery in Wutasi, Beijing, China. A team of Italian scientists described the remains of the famous castrato Farinelli, excavated in CE 2006 from a cemetery in Bologna, Italy, though his remains were unfortunately damaged due to water penetration of the burial plot. (Belcastro et al., 2011, 2014). The remains of the Lyon castrate and Nekht-Ankh were reexamined by the author to determine if modern paleopathological methods could elicit additional information about the effects of castration.

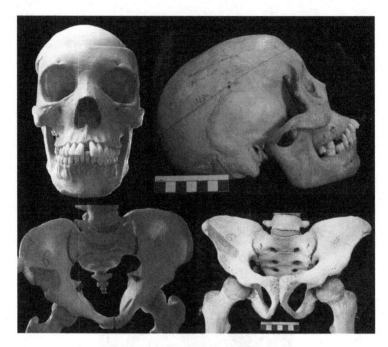

Figure 5.5 Clockwise from top left: Front and right lateral views of the skull and front and superior views of the pelvic girdle of the Lyon castrate. Writing on the right lateral side of the skull says "Eunuque negre, 20 ans env^{on} (?), Le Caire, 1894. Dr Lortet(?)" (Black eunuch, 20 years, Cairo [where this individual died and was autopsied], 1894. Dr Lortet [the doctor who brought the skeleton back to Lyon]). Source: Photo by author.

A comparison of these skeletons found similar results to earlier studies of human and animal castrates, but added the observations that the pelvic girdle formed masculine sex characteristics, though the ilia form unusual, flared shapes, and the skull takes on feminine or indeterminate sex characteristics, with strongly prognathic maxillae and strong, heavy mandibles overpowering the more delicate craniofacial region. In essence, castrates appear to belong physically between male and female and adult and child in skeletal development (Reusch, 2013a) (Fig. 5.5).

5.4 DETECTING CASTRATES WITHIN ARCHAEOLOGICAL POPULATIONS

Examinations of the skeletons of the Lyon castrate and Nekht-Ankh, along with comparisons to the Eng and Tandler and Grosz skeletons, have highlighted some distinct characteristics of castrate skeletons (Reusch, 2013a,b). These characteristics may aid in the detection of castrates both during excavation and in the laboratory, but one of the best ways of detecting castrates in large skeletal collections may be through the statistical analysis of their metrical data. The anthropometric measurements given by Wagenseil (Wagenseil, 1927, 1933) following Martin's (1914) standards (which use the same skeletal landmarks as osteometric measurements) were converted into osteometric measurements and added to the database of castrate skeletal measurements. Combined with data from complete skeletons derived from the FORDISC database (Ousley and Jantz, 2005), this allowed the separation of castrates from both males and females through the use of Linear and Mahalanobis Distance discriminant function analysis (Reusch, 2013a). This statistical method also clearly separated male, female, and castrated sheep from the Davis sample (Davis, 2000; Reusch, 2013a), making this method useful for detecting both human and animal castrates within archaeological collections.

5.5 CONCLUSIONS

While the lack of castrate skeletal material available to be examined might seem like an insurmountable challenge to a bioarchaeological examination of castration, this project actually gained a richer, more nuanced depiction of castrates through its need to develop information from multiple interdisciplinary sources of evidence. By studying historical accounts, castrates as physical and social individuals were highlighted, and the locations of castrate populations were mapped, allowing for the future detection of possible castrate burial places.

The lack of available skeletons also increased the need to understand historical interpretations of the physical body and the effects of castration on male bodies. It highlighted historical social prejudices toward castrates and the effects of personal bias on the interpretation of history. The need to rely on previously collected data also necessitated a closer mesh between anthropometric and osteometric data, giving new tools which can be used in other areas of anthropological research. The reworking of a useful statistical sexing tool, discriminant function analysis, to account for three sex groups (male, female, and castrate) allows intersex individuals to be pulled out from the wider population, making their detection easier. Further refinement of this method might allow for the separation of different intersex individuals from each other. This will not only aid human skeletal studies, but zooarchaeological ones as well, providing better methods of determining when castration in humans and animals began, and giving us a clearer picture of the past.

While the use of disparate datasets can be a daunting task, it has the potential to greatly expand our knowledge of subjects, giving unique insights into topics sometimes considered mundane or irrelevant. By combining art, humanities, social sciences, sciences, and medicine in this study, more knowledge about the lives of castrates was obtained than would have been possible from a study of only their skeletons, and new and different uses of tools were found which could have a great impact on anthropology and archaeology in the future.

ACKNOWLEDGMENTS

This project and paper would not have been possible without the generous contributions of time and effort by several individuals. First and foremost, Madeleine Mant and Alyson Holland, the organizers of the conference session and the editors of this volume, asked what it was possible to achieve with disparate datasets and brought together this fascinating group of papers which show a fantastic range of answers. Dr J.C. Neidhardt, the conservator and curator of the Testut Latarje Medical Anatomical Museum of (at the time) the University of Lyon, Lyon, France, granted permission to examine the remains of the Lyon castrate. Dr Karen Exell, former curator of Egypt and Sudan at the Manchester Museum, Manchester, England, initially granted permission to examine the Two Brothers mummies, and Dr Campbell Price, current curator of Egypt and the Sudan, kindly arranged for me to reexamine the mummies. Professor Richard Jantz of the University of Tennessee Knoxville provided access to the FORDISC database. Dr Beatrice Patzak of the Pathological Anatomical Museum of Vienna, Austria allowed me to examine records for traces of the Tandler and Grosz eunuch, which disappeared sometime after the initial CE 1909 publication. Several kind librarians from around the world scanned obscure papers and sent them to me, and I owe a great debt to the Google Books Gutenburg initiative, which has made available for free so many of the rare books necessary for the success of this project. I also had the generous support and assistance of members of my family and friends in reading, editing, and discussing both the thesis and this chapter. Caitlin Reusch-Zerr graciously assisted in the creation of the maps displayed in this chapter, making sure they were up to modern GIS mapping standards.

This project would not have been possible 10 years ago. The time, effort, and money that would have been required to visit all 10 or so of the institutions that hold the one or two remaining copies of some of these works would have been impossible for a graduate student or even an employed scholar who was not independently wealthy. In the ongoing effort to employ interdisciplinary methods to archaeological and anthropological practice, it is likely that the Internet and digital humanities will provide a major source of information in the future. Training for the location, use, and interpretation of digital sources should be a priority now for the benefit of the discipline in the future.

REFERENCES

Aristotle, 1984. The Complete Works of Aristotle: The Revised Oxford Translation. (J. Barnes, Trans.) Bollingen Series. Princeton University Press, Princeton, NJ.

Armitage, P.L., Clutton-Brock, J., 1976. A system for classification and description of the horn cores of cattle from archaeological sites. J. Archaeol. Sci. 3, 329–348.

Asher-Greve, J.M., 1997. The essential body: mesopotamian conceptions of the gendered body. Gender Hist. 9, 432–461.

Aucoin, M.W., Wassersug, R.J., 2006. The sexuality and social performance of androgen-deprived (castrated) men throughout history: implications for modern day cancer patients. Soc. Sci. Med. 63, 3162–3173.

Barbier, P., 1998. The World of the Castrati: The History of an Extraordinary Operatic Phenomenon, New ed. Souvenir Press Ltd., London.

Beard, M., 2012. The cult of the "Great Mother" in Imperial Rome. In: Brandt, J.R., Iddeng, J.W. (Eds.), Greek and Roman festivals. Oxford University Press, Oxford, pp. 323–362.

Belcastro, M.G., Todero, A., Fornaciari, G., Mariotti, V., 2011. Hyperostosis frontalis interna (HFI) and castration: the case of the famous singer Farinelli (1705–1782). J. Anat. 219, 632–637.

Belcastro, M.G., Mariotti, V., Bonfiglioli, B., Todero, A., Bocchini, G., Bettuzzi, M., et al., 2014. Dental status and 3D reconstruction of the malocclusion of the famous singer Farinelli (1705–1782). Int. J. Palaeopath. 7, 64–69.

Bi, H., Xiao, Q., 2009. Eunuchism of Imperial China from the perspective of world history. J. Cambridge Studies 4, 105–110.

Brett, M.A., Roberts, L.F., Johnson, T.W., Wassersug, R.J., 2007. Eunuchs in contemporary society: expectations, consequences, and adjustments to castration (part II). J. Sex. Med. 4, 946–955.

Briant, P., 2002. From Cyrus to Alexander: A History of the Persian Empire. Eisenbrauns, Winona Lake.

Bullough, V.L., 2002. Eunuchs in history and society. In: Tougher, S. (Ed.), Eunuchs in Antiquity and Beyond. Classical Press of Wales and Duckworth, London, pp. 1–17.

Coughlan, S., 2012. Breakthrough in world's oldest undeciphered writing [WWW Document]. BBC News, October 25, 2012. <http://www.bbc.com/news/business-19964786> (accessed 03.02.16).

Dahinten, S.L., Pucciarelli, H.M., 1986. Variations in sexual dimorphism in the skulls of rats subjected to malnutrition, castration, and treatment with gonadal hormones. Am. J. Phys. Anthropol. 71, 63–67.

Dalley, S., 2002. Evolution of gender in mesopotamian mythology and iconography with a possible explanation of ša rešen, the man with two heads. In: Parpola, S., Whiting, R.M. (Eds.), Sex and Gender in the Ancient Near East: Proceedings of the 47th Rencontre Assyriologique Internationale, Helsinki, July 2–6, 2001. Neo-Assyrian Text Corpus Project.

Davis, S.J.M., 2000. The effect of castration and age on the development of the Shetland sheep skeleton and a metric comparison between bones of males, females and castrates. J. Archaeol. Sci. 27, 373–390.

Doran, C., 2010. Chinese palace eunuchs: shadows of the emperor. Nebula 7, 11–26.

Dreger, A.D., 1998. Hermaphrodites and the Medical Invention of Sex. Harvard University Press, Cambridge, MA.

El-Cheikh, N.M., 2005. Servants at the gate: eunuchs at the Court of al-Muqtadir. J. Econ. Soc. Hist. Orie. 48, 234–252.

Engelstein, L., 1999. Castration and the Heavenly Kingdom: A Russian Folktale. Cornell University Press, Ithaca, NY.

Eng, J.T., Zhang, Q., Zhu, H., 2010. Skeletal effects of castration on two eunuchs of Ming China. Anthropol. Sci. 118, 107–116.

Fausto-Sterling, A., 2000. Sexing the Body: Gender Politics and the Construction of Sexuality. Basic Books, New York, NY.

Freitas, R., 2003. The eroticism of emasculation: confronting the Baroque body of the castrato. J. Musicol. 20, 196–249.

Gerbino, G., 2004. The quest for the soprano voice: castrati in Renaissance Italy. Stud. Music 33, 303–357.

Ghosh, P., 2015. DNA study finds London was ethnically diverse from start. BBC News, November 23, 2015. <http://www.bbc.com/news/science-environment-34809804> (accessed 03.02.16).

Greenfield, H.J., 2010. The secondary products revolution: the past, the present and the future. World Archaeol. 42, 29–54.

Hegarty, P.K., Mushtaq, I., Sebire, N.J., 2007. Natural history of testicular regression syndrome and consequences for clinical management. J. Pediatr. Urol. 3, 206–208.

Herdt, G.H. (Ed.), 1994. Third Sex, Third Gender: Beyond Sexual Dimorphism in Culture and History. Zone Books, New York, NY.

Hiort, O., 2002. Androgens and puberty. Best Pract. Res. Clin. Endocrinol. Metab. 16, 31–41.

Hiort, O., Holterhus, P.M., Drop, S., 2007. Normal and abnormal sex development. Best Pract. Res. Clin. Endocrinol. Metab. 21, vii–viii.

Hornblower, S., 2003. Panionios of Chios and Hermotimos of Pedasa (Hdt. 8. 104-6). In: Derow, P., Parker, R. (Eds.), Herodotus and His World: Essays from a Conference in Memory of George Forrest. Oxford University Press, Oxford, pp. 37–57.

Jay, J.W., 1993. Another side of Chinese eunuch history: castration, marriage, adoption, and burial. Can. J. Hist. 28, 459–478.

Jenkins, J.S., 1998. The voice of the castrato. Lancet 351, 1877–1880.

Jenkins, J.S., 2001. Long-term consequences of castration in men. J. Clin. Endocr. Metab. 86, 1844.

Kadish, G.E., 1969. Eunuchs in Ancient Egypt? In: Kadish, G.E. (Ed.), Studies in Honour of J. A. Wilson. University of Chicago Press, Chicago, IL, pp. 55–62.

Kenny, A.M., Raisz, L.G., 2003. Androgens and bone. In: Bagatell, C.J., Bremner, W.J. (Eds.), Androgens in Health and Disease. Humana Press, Totowa, NJ, pp. 221–232.

Koch, W., 1921. Über die russisch-rumänische kastratensekte der Skopzen. Ver. Kreigs Konstitutionspathol. 7, 1–39.

Krimmer, E., 2005. "Eviva il Coltello"? The castrato singer in eighteenth-century German literature and culture. PMLA 120, 1543–1559.

Kutcher, N.A., 2010. Unspoken collusions: the empowerment of Yuanming yuan eunuchs in the Qianlong Period. Harvard J. Asait. Stud. 70, 449–495.

Lane, C., 1978. Christian Religion in the Soviet Union: A Sociological Study. SUNY Press, Albany, NJ.

Leick, G., 2003. Sex and Eroticism in Mesopotamian Literature. Routledge, London.

Llewellyn-Jones, L., 2002. Eunuchs and the Royal Harem in Achaemenid Persia (599-331 B.C.). In: Tougher, S. (Ed.), Eunuchs in Antiquity and Beyond. Classical Press of Wales and Duckworth, London, pp. 19–49.

Lortet, L.-C., 1896. Allongment des Membres Infèrieurs du a la Castration. Arch. d'Anthropol. Crim. 64, 361–364.

Magie, D., 1924. (Trans.) Scriptores Historiae Augustae. William Heinemann, London.

Marmon, S.E., 1995. Eunuchs and Sacred Boundaries in Islamic Society. Oxford University Press, Oxford.

Martin, R., 1914. Lehrbuch der Anthropologie in systematischer Darstellung: mit besonderer Berücksichtigung der anthropologischen Methoden für Studierende Ärzte und Forschungsreisende. G. Fischer, Jena.

Matthews, D., 1994. The secular and Religious Roles of the Eunuch in Assyria. Université de Montréal, Montréal (unpublished MA thesis).

Milner, A., 1973. The sacred capons. Music. Times 114, 250–252.

Mitamura, T., 1970. Chinese Eunuchs: The Structure of Intimate Politics. C.E. Tuttle Co, Rutland.

Mukherjee, J.B., 1980. Castration—a means of induction into the Hijirah group of the eunuch community in India. Am. J. Foren. Med. Path. 1, 61–65.

Murray, M.A., 1910. The Tomb of Two Brothers. Sherratt & Hughes, Manchester.

Nanda, S., 1999. Neither Man Nor Woman: The Hijras of India. Wadsworth Publishing Co, Belmont, CA.

Orton, D.C., 2014. Secondary products and the "secondary products revolution". In: Smith, C. (Ed.), Encyclopedia of Global Archaeology. Springer, New York, NY, pp. 6541–6547.

Ousley, S.D., Jantz, R.L., 2005. FORDISC 3.0 Personal Computer Forensic Discriminant Functions. University of Tennessee, Knoxville, TN.

Patterson, O., 1982. The ultimate slave. In: Patterson, O. (Ed.), Slavery and Social Death: A Comparative Study. Harvard University Press, Cambridge, MA, pp. 299–333.

Pittard, E., 1934. La castration chez l'homme et les modifications morphologiques qu'elle entraîne. Recherches sur les adeptes d'une secte d'eunuques mystiques. Les Skoptzy. Masson et Cie, Paris.

Plymate, S., 2003. Hypogonadism in Men: An Overview. In: Bagatell, C.J., Bremner, W.J. (Eds.), Androgens in Health and Disease. Humana Press, Totowa, NJ, pp. 45–76.

Potter, J., 2007. The tenor–castrato connection, 1760–1860. Early Music 35, 97–112.

Preston, L.W., 1987. A right to exist: eunuchs and the state in nineteenth-century India. Mod. Asian Stud. 21, 371–387.

Quigley, C.A., Bellis, A.D., Marschke, K.B., El-Awady, M.K., Wilson, E.M., French, F.S., 1995. Androgen receptor defects: historical, clinical, and molecular perspectives. Endocr. Rev. 16, 271–321.

Reis, E., 2005. Impossible hermaphrodites: intersex in America, 1620-1960. J. Am. Hist. 92, 411–441.

Reusch, K., 2013a. "That Which Was Missing": The Archaeology of Castration. University of Oxford, Oxford (unpublished PhD dissertation). Available either through the Oxford University Research Archive <http://ora.ox.ac.uk/objects/uuid:b8118fe7-67cb-4610-9823-b0242dfe900a> or by request to the author via email (k.l.reusch@gmail.com) or academia.edu <https://www.academia.edu/9717531/_That_Which_Was_Missing_The_Archaeology_of_Castration>.

Reusch, K., 2013b. Raised voices: the archaeology of castration. In: Tracy, L. (Ed.), Castration and Culture in the Middle Ages. D.S. Brewer, Cambridge, MA, pp. 29–47.

Ringrose, K.M., 1994. Living in the shadows: eunuchs and gender in Byzantium. In: Herdt, G. (Ed.), Third Sex, Third Gender: Beyond Sexual Dimorphism in Culture and History. Zone Books, New York, NY, pp. 85–110.

Ringrose, K.M., 1999. Passing the test of sanctity: denial of sexuality and involuntary castration. In: James, L. (Ed.), Desire and Denial in Byzantium. Ashgate/Variorum, Aldershot, pp. 123–137.

Ringrose, K.M., 2003. The Perfect Servant: Eunuchs and the Social Construction of Gender in Byzantium. University of Chicago Press, Chicago, IL.

Rosselli, J., 1988. The castrati as a professional group and a social phenomenon, 1550-1850. Acta Musicol. 60, 143–179.

Scholz, P.O., 2001. Eunuchs and Castrati: A Cultural History. Markus Wiener Publishers, Princeton, NJ.

Segal, R., 2001. Islam's Black Slaves: The Other Black Diaspora. Farrar, Straus and Giroux, New York, NY.

Sherratt, A., 1983. The secondary exploitation of animals in the Old World. World Archaeol. 15, 90–104.

Siddall, L.R., 2007. A re-examination of the Title ša reši in the Neo-Assyrian Period. In: Azize, J., Weeks, N. (Eds.), Gilgameš and the World of Assyria: Proceedings of the Conference Held at Mandelbaum House, the University of Sydney, July 21–23, 2004. Peeters Publishers, Leuven, pp. 225–240.

Tadmor, H., 1983. Rab-saris and Rab-shakeh in 2 Kings 18. In: Meyers, C.L., O'Connor, M. (Eds.), The Word of the Lord Shall Go Forth: Essays in Honor of David Noel Freedman in Celebration of His Sixtieth Birthday. Eisenbrauns, Philadelphia, PA, pp. 279–285.

Tandler, J., Grosz, S., 1910. Über den Einfluss der Kastration auf den Organismus II. Die Skopzen. Arch. Entwickl. Mech. Org. 28, 236–253.

Tandler, J., Grosz, S., 1909. Über den Einfluss der Kastration auf den Organismus I. Beschreibung eines Eunuchen skeletes. Arch. Entwickl. Mech. Org. 27, 35–45.

Taylor, G., 2002. Castration: An Abbreviated History of Western Manhood. Routledge, New York, NY.

Tougher, S., 1997. Byzantine eunuchs: an overview, with special reference to their creation and origin. In: James, L. (Ed.), Women, Men, and Eunuchs: Gender in Byzantium. Routledge, London, pp. 168–199.

Tougher, S. (Ed.), 2002. Eunuchs in Antiquity and Beyond. Classical Press of Wales and Duckworth, London.

Tougher, S., 2008. The Eunuch in Byzantine History and Society. Routledge, London.

Tougher, S., 2013. The aesthetics of castration: the beauty of roman eunuchs. In: Tracy, L. (Ed.), Castration and Culture in the Middle Ages. Boydell & Brewer, Cambridge, MA, pp. 48–72.

Tsai, S.H., 1996. The Eunuchs in the Ming Dynasty. SUNY Press, Albany, NJ.

Vanderschueren, D., Boonen, S., Bouillon, R., 1998. Action of androgens versus estrogens in male skeletal homeostasis. Bone 23, 391–394.

Vermaseren, M.J., 1977. Cybele and Attis: The Myth and the Cult, First Ed. Thames & Hudson Ltd, London.

Vinci, G., Anjot, M.-N., Trivin, C., Lottmann, H., Brauner, R., McElreavey, K., 2004. An analysis of the genetic factors involved in testicular descent in a cohort of 14 male patients with anorchia. J. Clin. Endocr. Metab. 89, 6282–6285.

von Bayern, R., 1923. Reiseerinnerungen aus dem Süd-Osten Europas und dem Orient. Kösel & Pustet, München.

Wagenseil, F., 1927. Beiträge zur Kenntnis der Kastrationsfolgen und des Eunchoidismus beim Mann. Z. Morphol. Anthropol. 26, 264–304.

Wagenseil, F., 1933. Chinesische Eunuchen. (Zugleich ein Beitrag zur Kenntnis der Kastrationsfolgen und der rassialen und körperbaulichen Bedeutung der anthropologischen Merkmale). Z. Morphol. Anthropol. 32, 415–468.

Ware, R.T., 2011. Slavery in Islamic Africa, 1400-1800. In: Eltis, D., Engerman, L.S. (Eds.), The Cambridge World History of Slavery: AD 1420-AD 1804. Cambridge University Press, Cambridge, MA, pp. 47–80.

Wilson, J.D., Roehrborn, C., 1999. Long-term consequences of castration in men: lessons from the Skoptzy and the eunuchs of the Chinese and Ottoman courts. J. Clin. Endocr. Metab 84, 4324–4331.

Winters, S.J., Clark, B.J., 2003. Testosterone synthesis, transport and metabolism. In: Bagatell, C.J., Bremner, W.J. (Eds.), Androgens in Health and Disease. Humana Press, Totowa, NJ, pp. 3–22.

CHAPTER 6

Hunting for Pathogens: Ancient DNA and the Historical Record

S. Marciniak
Department of Anthropology, McMaster University, Hamilton, ON, Canada

The bioarchaeological investigation of disease benefits from an interdisciplinary approach because the disease process itself is multifaceted; its expression is responsive to the environment, and is influenced by human activity. Ancient DNA is a powerful research tool, capable of addressing diverse questions surrounding the origin, distribution, susceptibility, or evolutionary changes of a pathogen and the disease it may cause (eg, Devault et al., 2014a; Spigelman et al., 2015; Wagner et al., 2014). Upon integration with other lines of evidence such as ancient literary texts, archaeological data, or skeletal analyses, the experience of disease in antiquity may be illuminated.

The integration of ancient DNA analysis in a bioarchaeological study typically relies on selecting skeletal samples associated with presumed pathogens. Disease may be identified by diagnostic skeletal changes (eg, *facies leprosa* indicative of leprosy; Andersen and Manchester, 1992), catastrophic assemblages from epidemics or plagues connected to an infectious agent (eg, *Yersinia pestis* and the Black Death; Bos et al., 2011; Drancourt et al., 1998), or literary evidence describing symptomology in the wake of mass mortality (eg, Plague of Athens; Page, 1953). Such exclusive association is rare in the archaeological record due to the Osteological Paradox: (1) few infectious diseases induce skeletal responses, as only 5−20% of individuals manifest pathological changes (Ortner, 2008; Roberts and Manchester, 2005; Steinbock, 1976); (2) chronic or long-term infections (eg, tuberculosis, leprosy) are predominant, whereas acute infections of rapid mortality or spontaneous recovery (eg, bubonic plague, malaria) leave no skeletal traces (Roberts and Manchester, 2005; Steinbock, 1976); and (3) susceptibility to disease (heterogeneity and frailty)

Beyond the Bones. DOI: http://dx.doi.org/10.1016/B978-0-12-804601-2.00006-5

means that there is individual variability in responses to infection (Wood et al., 1992; Wright and Yoder, 2003).

This chapter presents a scenario exploring infectious diseases in three Imperial Roman necropoleis (ancient cemeteries) (Italy, 1st–4th century CE), utilizing disparate datasets: ancient DNA analysis of skeletal remains, complemented by literary and archaeological evidence.

6.1 EXPLORING DISEASE IN IMPERIAL ROMAN NECROPOLEIS

The cemeteries of Vagnari (2nd–4th century CE; see Prowse et al., 2010; Small, 2011, 2014), Velia (1st–2nd century CE; see Craig et al., 2009; Crowe et al., 2010; Fiammenghi, 2003), and Isola Sacra (associated with Portus Romae) (1st–3rd century CE; see Bondioli et al., 1995; Prowse et al., 2005, 2007) are geographically disparate necropoleis in Italy. The individuals buried at Vagnari likely represent a workforce associated with a rural inland estate far from urban centers (Prowse et al., 2014; Small, 2011, 2014), while Velia and Portus Romae were important port cities and maritime trading centers, closely connected to the Roman capital (Craig et al., 2009; Keay and Paroli, 2011; Prowse et al., 2007). Similar to other skeletal assemblages indicating health stressors across Roman Italy (Cucina et al., 2006; Eckardt, 2010; Facchini et al., 2004; Killgrove, 2010), there is skeletal evidence of nonspecific stressors (eg, linear enamel hypoplasias, cribra orbitalia, porotic hyperostosis) at Vagnari (Prowse et al., 2014), Isola Sacra (Gowland and Garnsey, 2010), and Velia (Beauchesne, 2012). In such contexts, ancient DNA facilitates the identification of disease-associated pathogens since it is difficult to diagnose specific diseases based solely upon skeletal changes.

To comprehensively investigate morbidity and mortality within these Imperial period assemblages, it is necessary to apply an approach mentioned by Killgrove (2014) that systematically considers multiple factors associated with a dynamic disease-scape, such as malnutrition, sanitation and hygiene, social status, urbanization, and infrastructure as well as cocirculating and coinfecting pathogens. The objectives of the necropoleis project outlined in this chapter are twofold: (1) assess candidate pathogens through metagenomic "shotgun" sequencing of the entire microbial DNA as a means to infer pathogen presence; and (2) contextualize the molecular data using archaeological evidence related to disease ecology at each site and evaluate the degree to which selected ancient literary texts enable inferences of prospective diseases beyond the Roman capital to other parts of Roman Italy. The goal is to explore factors mitigating or proliferating disease in diverse assemblages of the Imperial Roman period using a framework that emphasizes the multifactorial pathways of disease.

6.2 CHARACTERIZING ANCIENT PATHOGENS

6.2.1 Ancient DNA and Pathogen Detection

For the Roman necropoleis, a single tooth was selected from 20 adult individuals in each necropolis (for a total of 60 teeth) as part of a large-scale screening approach to maximize the detection of pathogens alongside the range of environmental, commensal, and contaminant microorganisms within individual metagenomes. Shotgun sequencing was applied as a screening method to evaluate whether human pathogens, based on Roman historical and bioarchaeological evidence, are identifiable in the metagenomic datasets generated from the Roman necropoleis samples, rather than as a tool for the definitive identification of pathogens.

In integrating ancient DNA in bioarchaeological studies, there are a number of issues that merit consideration. Primarily, ancient DNA exhibits signatures of molecular and chemical degradation alongside idiosyncratic preservation (intra- and inter-specimen variability), resulting in an abundance of damaged short DNA fragments (on average 30–60 base pairs or bp) compared to modern biological DNA (see reviews by Hofreiter et al., 2014; Molak and Ho, 2011). These factors directly affect the complexity of DNA constituents, which predominantly contain environmental (eg, soil, sediment, or macroorganisms, such as plants or fungi), modern contaminant, and non-target DNA, with a low endogenous content (eg, 0–5%) (Burbano et al., 2010; Carpenter et al., 2013; Pääbo et al., 2004). There are notable exceptions, however, where well-preserved genomic data are retrievable, such as permafrost specimens (see Bellemain et al., 2013; Legendre et al., 2014). The challenge is that the minute pathogen DNA fraction in human bones and teeth is embedded within the entirety of a dynamic DNA "pool," and this poses a significant obstacle to resolving historical pathogen presence.

When applying ancient DNA methodologies in a context such as the Roman necropoleis, where disease-associated pathogens are unknown, it is critical to consider the appropriate specimen to enable broad-spectrum detection of blood-borne pathogens. Teeth are considered optimum substrates—particularly subsamples of the root or recovering dental pulp—due to substantial vascularization and increased protection from molecular degradation, whereas bone is a less ideal substrate, as it can absorb significant amounts of contaminant DNA from the burial environment (Adler et al., 2011; Drancourt et al., 1998; Higgins and Austin, 2013).

Metagenomic "shotgun" sequencing or sequencing without the selection of targets (ie, loci, genes, genomes) is useful when there is no knowledge of a presumed disease and in consideration of the confounding host and environmental factors (eg, host susceptibility, heterogeneity of risk) contributing to the expression of disease (Devault et al., 2014b; Orlando et al., 2015; Warinner et al., 2015). Shotgun sequencing demonstrates success in ancient DNA research, such as Kay et al. (2014) obtaining 6.5-fold coverage of a *Brucella melitensis* genome from the calcified nodule of a medieval specimen. The approach is the least biased, compared to amplicon sequencing (16S rRNA genes) or targeted capture strategies (these require a presumed pathogen), and is the most comprehensive means of characterizing the entire microbial DNA content of a sample (Devault et al., 2014b; Warinner et al., 2015; Whatmore, 2014). A caveat with shotgun sequencing is that low abundant human pathogens are often undetectable within these substantial metagenomic datasets (eg, comprising less than 0.08% of sequence reads in Devault et al., 2014b) and it remains cost-prohibitive to deeply sequence samples for diagnostic pathogen identification (defined as greater than $30 \times$ for meaningful genome coverage).

6.2.2 Metagenomic Pathogen Screening From the Necropoleis

As noted by Scheidel (2009), the uncertainties surrounding the knowledge of health and disease in ancient Rome enables diverse scenarios to be constructed from multiple evidentiary sources. In this sense, the framework applied to prioritize candidate disease-associated pathogens in Velia, Vagnari, and Portus Romae relies on historical reasoning and drawing contextually relevant factors from the disparate sources.

It is beyond the scope of this chapter to comprehensively discuss the bioinformatic processing of the Roman sequence data and the specific metagenomic results (eg, microbial diversity and taxa abundance, data authentication). Samples were processed at the McMaster Ancient DNA Centre (Hamilton, ON, Canada), with physically separated ancient DNA and modern laboratory facilities. DNA was extracted using a protocol modified from Schwarz et al. (2009) and libraries suitable for sequencing on the Illumina HiSeq 1500 platform (75 bp paired-end read chemistry) (Illumina, San Diego, CA, United States) were prepared with modifications in previously published protocols (Kircher et al., 2012; Meyer and Kircher, 2010). Raw sequence reads were trimmed to remove residual adaptors and then merged using SeqPrep (St. John, 2011).

Briefly, 180,000 to 8,000,000 raw (unprocessed) DNA reads were generated across the Roman samples and the processed metagenomic datasets varied from 500,000 to 4,000,000 sequence reads across the 60 Roman libraries (one for each tooth sample). Negative controls (ie, extraction blanks) were processed alongside the Roman libraries and demonstrate low abundance bacterial sequences (less than 300 reads).

To establish that the retrieved ancient DNA is authentic, protocols are proposed to prevent and detect contamination (eg, Cooper and Poinar, 2000), including separate ancient and modern DNA laboratories, unique nucleotide damage patterns associated with ancient specimens (cytosine deamination near the 5′ ends of fragments), and appropriate molecular behavior (the degradation of DNA into an abundance of short fragments compared to few long fragments) (see Briggs et al., 2009; Brotherton et al., 2007; Lindahl, 1993). Bioinformatic estimates of contamination (eg, Ginolhac et al., 2011; Skoglund et al., 2014) require mapping the sequences to a reference (eg, a specific pathogen genome or genes), which is not always possible with metagenomic data (as mentioned by Warinner et al., 2015). This is observed in the Roman data discussed here, with a low number of reads (and subsequent low coverage) when mapping to candidate human pathogen genes.

The onus is on the researcher to critically analyze the project design and incorporate relevant criteria to evaluate the validity of the sequence data (Gilbert et al., 2005). Accordingly, the proportion of reads from the Roman samples mapping (matching) to the human mitochondrial genome (revised Cambridge Reference Sequence) (as a proxy for inferring authenticity) varied from 0.003% to 1.2%, and the sequences demonstrate signatures of authentic and highly degraded ancient DNA as evidenced by higher rates of deamination (C to T and G to A transitions near the 5′ and 3′ ends of fragments, respectively), read length distributions indicating the predominance of short DNA sequences (24−60 bp), and characteristic fragmentation patterns.

The Roman shotgun data were processed to identify taxonomic assignments by comparison to a nucleotide sequence database (blastn-megablast, v.2.2.29) (Altschul et al., 1990). Each BLAST (Basic Local Alignment Search Tool) output was parsed using MEGAN4 (MEtaGenome ANalyzer, v.4.70.4) in order to assign a taxon (Huson et al., 2007). The results of the MEGAN4 output demonstrate extensive metagenomic diversity, capable of Family- to Species-level characterization, with a range of 3−30% of reads taxonomically identifiable across all samples. The Bacteria taxon is the most predominant in the number of assigned reads, followed by the Eukaryota (eg, Fungi, Viridiplantae) and Hominoidea taxa. Comparisons of the taxonomic distributions across the samples depended on the resolution of the data (ie, number of reads taxonomically identified to the Genus or Species level, number of unassigned reads), and ranges from soil organisms characteristic of salt/marsh environments (eg, *Desulfovibrio* spp., *Aeromonas* spp.), to organisms of the human microbiome (eg, skin and gut flora, such as *Propionibacterium*) and pathogenic components (eg, periodontal disease agents, such as *Tannerella forsythia*). Human-only pathogens are present in low abundance in the Roman metagenomic dataset, varying from 0.03% to 3% (or 0.9% on average) of taxonomically identifiable sequence reads. The presumptive pathogens identified and selected as candidates for further analysis included: *Mycobacterium tuberculosis*, *Mycobacterium leprae*, *Clostridium botulinum*, and *Clostridium tetani*.

There are challenges in using taxonomic assignments as a means to identify candidate pathogens from the necropoleis of Velia, Vagnari, and Isola Sacra. Methodologically, this confidence threshold relates to a key parameter of MEGAN functionality, the ability to assign short reads (less than 50 bp) to a taxonomic level (Huson et al., 2007). The low number of human pathogen taxa observed with the Roman metagenomic data is partly attributed to the short read lengths, ultimately producing fewer taxa assignments, thereby underpredicting the number of reads associated with a taxa and actual metagenomic content (Huson et al., 2007). MEGAN's computational approach emphasizes sensitivity, but the conservative measure of taxon identification limits the use of the Roman metagenomic dataset to definitively include or exclude the presence of specific disease-associated pathogens. This means that a particular taxon assignment is not irrefutable evidence of a target's presence, nor is the absence of pathogen DNA certain when not identified taxonomically. The degree to which any pathogen is identified in the metagenomic dataset requires examination of the reads that are the basis of its taxonomic assignment. Alignments and mapping to the presumed pathogen genome (or genes) are also important to identify the particular genomic regions used to "call" the taxonomic identification.

In this sense, although pathogen candidates are identifiable from the shotgun data, it is unknowable which pathogens have been undetected or underrepresented with this molecular strategy. The sequence depth of one million reads per sample is insufficient to fully characterize the necropoleis samples' genomic composition; however, without previous molecular work on these ancient Roman samples, shotgun sequencing provides a preliminary assessment of predominant taxa abundance and diversity, with indications of disease-associated pathogens present to later target via hybridization capture (ie, the sequestration of DNA via known sequence probes or "baits"). To address the challenges of implementing a shotgun sequencing strategy using previously uncharacterized ancient samples to evaluate pathogen presence, it is critical to further refine the nosological context by identifying contextually relevant diseases presumed to be present in ancient Rome to evaluate applicability within the necropoleis under study, and establishing the epidemiological environment at the sites.

6.2.3 Integrating Metagenomic Data With the Historical Record
6.2.3.1 Literary Texts and Disease-Associated Pathogens
The use of ancient written sources presents a unique set of challenges in reconstructing disease presence in the past, since texts represent a specific context of experiencing and understanding disease (Leven, 2004; Rosenberg, 1992). From the available range of ancient Greek and Roman literary evidence, scholars infer circulating diseases within the Roman world to include tuberculosis, typhoid fever, malaria, leprosy, gastroenteritis, cholera, dysentery, syphilis, herpes, and brucellosis (Grmek, 1989; Nutton, 2004; Sallares, 2002; Scheidel, 2003, 2009);

however, it is critical to recognize the relationship between the humoral theory of the Hippocratic tradition during this time and the practice of retrospective diagnoses.

Within humoral theory, there were no unique causal explanations for disease and the focus was on discovering the underlying humoral imbalance in the individual that produced the observed illness (Grmek, 1989; Nutton, 2004). The translation of these ancient descriptions into diagnosed "named diseases" inadvertently imposes contemporary knowledge about diseases upon the past (Grmek, 1989; Mitchell, 2011; Nutton, 2004). For example, the use of "lepra" (scaly, thickened skin) in the Hippocratic tradition indicates a variety of benign dermato-logical conditions, such as psoriasis or eczema, not solely *Mycobacterium leprae*, as it is understood today (Nutton, 2004). This means a variety of conditions or diseases may have been associated with these descriptions; accordingly, it was necessary to integrate an approach that did not focus on establishing "named diseases" from these texts, but evaluated the picture of disease expression (or a syndromic approach) proposed by Muramoto (2014) by applying contemporary epidemiological concepts (ie, factors proliferating or mitigating disease).

Within the retrospective interpretation of diseases, it is also critical to be aware of the particularities related to the Roman context. The literary record itself is highly fragmentary with a scarcity of documen-tation on chronic diseases and epidemic outbreaks during the Late Republican and Imperial periods as noted by Scheidel (2009) where only 15 epidemics were recorded from the 2nd century BCE to the 8th century CE. The practice of ancient authors copying from earlier texts without acknowledging predecessors also complicates assessment of whether descriptions were developed with firsthand knowledge of the disease (Grmek, 1989; Mitchell, 2011; Nutton, 2004). These factors necessitate emphasis on the Roman context of experiencing and under-standing disease as shown by the literary evidence. Due to an absence of specific written evidence (eg, medical texts, personal accounts) for the necropoleis of Vagnari, Velia, and Isola Sacra, select ancient texts are used to draw inferences of the disease experience at a given time (defined as nosology, by Grmek, 1989) in the broad context of the Imperial period. Translated and original versions of ancient Greek and Roman medical texts associated with the Late Republic to Imperial periods used in this study included: (1) works of the Hippocratic Corpus (see Adams, 1891; Jouanna, 1999); (2) writings of the physician Galen (see Kühn, 1825); (3) Pliny the Elder (see Rackham, 1938); and (4) Celsus (see Collier, 1831).

In this sense the picture of disease is framed by the characterization of the Roman capital as similar to premodern urban societies (eg, preindustrial London) or a contemporary third world country (Dyson, 2010; Nutton, 2004; Scheidel, 2009), in order to facilitate the presumptive association of contextually relevant diseases, such as chronic infections (eg, tuberculosis, leprosy, syphilis), acute diseases (eg, smallpox, cholera), and opportunistic infections (eg, gastroenteritis attributed to *Salmonella* spp., *Staphylococcus* spp.) (eg, Grmek, 1989; Nutton, 2004; Scheidel, 2003, 2009). The inferences of infectious and parasitic diseases as the predominant agents in the pathogen pool of the Roman Empire are viewed as outcomes of a densely urbanized context, complicated by poor nutrition, crowded conditions, "unsanitary" practices (eg, improper corpse disposal, ineffective sewage systems), and environmental influences (eg, proximity to the Tiber River, flood frequency) (Dyson, 2010; Gowland and Garnsey, 2010; Scheidel, 2003, 2009). Descriptions drawn from not only medical texts, but also Roman practices of food preparation, animal husbandry, farming, or other daily activities may further outline the scope of disease-associated pathogens (most applicable for the rural estate of Vagnari), rather than those solely associated with preurban landscapes.

However, a complication with integrating the Roman metagenomic data in consideration of the historical record is that the geographic distribution of diseases is unknown within the Empire. References within the literary record are also restricted to specific locations, such as the Roman capital; while the Hippocratic Corpus is geographically confined to Thessaly and northern Greece, documenting selected cases of interest (Jouanna, 1999). This is a limiting factor in attempting to explore the seasonality or spatial range of morbidity or mortality associated with disease, particularly for the sites of Velia, Vagnari, and Portus Romae. Hippocrates' "Aphorisms" (III.XX–XXIII) (Adams, 1891) indicates specific diseases were exacerbated at particular times, such as continued, ardent, and tertian fevers in the summer or irregular fevers, dropsy, and phthisis in autumn. Inferences may be drawn from this text regarding seasonality of symptoms associated with descriptions of diseases; however, the coastal locations of Velia and Portus Romae, and the rural location of Vagnari further create a dynamic epidemiological environment due to diverse pathogen reservoirs and related human risk of exposure. Accordingly, the explanatory framework provides a picture of presumed diseases associated with life in the Roman Empire, but it is critical to consider the context from which these interpretations are based, as the conditions creating the pathogen pool in the Roman capital are not equivalent to the forces contributing to the pathogen burden at Vagnari, Velia, and Portus Romae.

Broad-based generalizations about the disease-scape in ancient Rome drawn from the literary record provide a picture from which to make inferences relating to the populations of Velia, Portus Romae, and Vagnari, although it is recognized that disease distribution was likely extremely heterogeneous. Going beyond generalized conclusions relating to the presence of diseases associated with a metropolitan environment is challenging for the rural and suburban Roman Italian populations. However, building the nosological context requires additional data from archaeological evidence related to disease ecology and is beneficial in refining the influences on pathogen exposure and disease expression.

6.2.3.2 Archaeological Data and the Disease-Scape

Archaeological evidence for human-modified landscapes and disease ecology is evaluated to frame potential exposure to pathogens within the necropoleis studied. The application of ecosocial epidemiological theory (Krieger, 2011) as part of an ecosystem approach to health (Waltner-Toews, 2001) creates a framework for the identification of factors potentially proliferating or limiting disease within Velia, Vagnari, and Portus Romae. Krieger's (2011, p. 215) concept of the "lived experience of disease" also guided the identification of ecological factors potentially affecting the retrospective burden of disease in these populations. Drawing from these frameworks, critical ecological components affecting the proliferation of disease(s) and causative agents were evaluated as the following: climate; landscape (type of soil or sediment, types of vegetation); geomorphology (topography changes, coastline formations); water bodies (lagoons, swamps, lakes); and extreme events (flooding, periods of aridity). This evidence was then applied in inferring disease ecology and the sustainability of pathogen transmission or survival at the local and regional scales.

The manifestation of disease is further structured within socio-cultural and political realms (Krieger, 2008) and, accordingly, the evaluation of human—environment interactions considered the impact of anthropogenic processes (eg, urbanization, agricultural practices, construction activities, trade, and migration) as active modifiers of disease ecology and the resultant disease burden (Krieger, 2011). In evaluating human agency as broadly modifying the pathogen pool within ancient Rome and the necropoleis in particular, a number of inferences were drawn from current epidemiological knowledge regarding disease transmission and sustainability in preurban landscapes (eg, population density, public infrastructure, human mobility). Integrating aspects of the paleoenvironment alongside evidence of human activities facilitates the reconstruction of a snapshot of the dynamic disease pool associated with the epidemiological environments of Velia, Vagnari, and Portus Romae at a given moment in historical time.

In using paleoenvironmental data from Vagnari, Velia, and Portus Romae, as well as the Mediterranean region to draw inferences on the factors proliferating or mitigating potential disease-associated patho-gens, there is dynamic potential in each environment to sustain pathogens; however, the ability of local ecosystems to modulate pathogen presence and exposure is not fully discernible solely through the archaeological record. Mediterranean pollen records indicate a warm and dry climate, typifying the current subtropical climate and landscape of indented coastlines, valleys, forests (coastal and woodland), and shrubland (Grove and Rackham, 2001; Sadori et al., 2011). However, it is only possible to broadly interpret the subtropical Roman Italian environment as *capable* of supporting vector-borne and parasitic diseases typically associated with such subtropical regions (WHO, 2015). Although the available paleoenvironmental evidence from Velia, Portus Romae, and Vagnari is variable, there remains the potential to evaluate the known and unknown factors contributing to local disease ecology.

At the scale of Vagnari, Velia, and Portus Romae, paleoen-vironmental data frame the conditions of the ancient environments within which individuals survived and thrived. The geographic distribution of pathogens within these ancient environments is affected by the landscape where the coastal geomorphology of Velia (cliffs, dunes, marshes, and bays; Amato et al., 2010) and Portus Romae (marshes, hills, dunes, and coastal woodlands; Di Rita et al., 2010; Keay and Paroli, 2011) contrast to inland Vagnari (lowland hills, river valley; Small, 2011, 2014), thereby highlighting the potential for heterogeneous distribution of pathogen reservoirs. For example, within Portus Romae the gradual and seasonal desiccation of a lagoon and marsh has consequences for vector colonization of surface pools (Di Rita et al., 2010; Keay and Paroli, 2011). The effect of extreme climatic events, such as flooding, affects the capability of public infrastructure and exacerbates infectious diseases (Bissell, 1983; Ivers and Ryan, 2006). For example, Portus Romae is in close proximity to the Tiber River with its record of recurrent floods (5th century BCE to 4th century CE) (Aldrete, 2007; Keay and Paroli, 2011), while the stratigraphy at Velia indicates flood events through sedimentation of alluvial deposits (Amato et al., 2010; Ruello, 2008). Although the paleoenvironmental evidence is limited among the sites, each merits evaluation regarding local disease ecology and the potential impact on the distribution of disease-associated pathogens. The integration of metagenomic data identifying candidate pathogens for each site, alongside explanatory frameworks of disease in the Imperial period, provides a means to contextualize the manifestation of these forces in the specific paleoenvironments of Velia, Vagnari, and Portus Romae.

Proxies of the causal pathways behind disease exposure and susceptibility (eg, population density, infrastructure, scale of urbanization, biocultural environment), as drawn from the Roman historical record and contemporary epidemiological knowledge, are integrated as a means to infer the influence of human activity on disease distribution at each site. The absence of demographic information for Velia, Portus Romae, and Vagnari limits inferences regarding transmission and survival of infectious diseases in suburban and rural contexts. Infrastructure is a critical determinant of population health, particularly the efficacy of Roman aqueducts and sewage systems in providing clean water while removing waste. The overflow from public basins and fountains is argued to contribute to surface cesspools of gastroenteritis, dysentery, cholera, and helminth infections (Scheidel, 2003, 2009; Scobie, 1986). For example, the proximity of residences to aqueducts in Portus Romae (Keay and Paroli, 2011), the terrace system in Velia (Amato et al., 2010), and the water-filled ravine that ran through Vagnari (Small, 2011) raise the issue of the potential for seepage or surface pools alongside flat stretches of land (Keiser et al., 2005). Similarly, the construction of buildings or residences (single or multistorey) may indicate the number of inhabitants, which relates to the potential for the communicability of disease. The distribution of such residential complexes, industrial and ceremonial buildings further contributes to varied patterns of disease.

Economic and political activities as outgrowths of urbanization during the Imperial period are significant in assessing the potential influence on pathogen burden. Maritime trade and immigration are capable of introducing novel pathogens into the population (Killgrove, 2014; Prowse et al., 2007; Scheidel, 2009), which relate to the sustainability of pathogen pools in the port cities of Velia and Portus Romae. The identification of nonlocal individuals at the sites of Vagnari (Prowse et al., 2010) and Portus Romae (Prowse et al., 2007) through isotopic or ancient DNA analysis is critical to address the distribution of disease among the inhabitants. The broad range of factors associated with servicing a growing Empire, such as irrigation canals as part of agricultural practices, road-building to expand connections among cities, and deforestation to harvest wood/timber potentially affect the frequency of human encounters with pathogen reservoirs (Sutherst, 2004; Yasuoka and Levins, 2007). For example, the Via Portuensis (linking Rome and Portus Romae) was constructed with small stone layers potentially proliferating the longevity of standing water (Keay and Paroli, 2011). The construction, frequency, and manner of maintenance for public infrastructure directly influence the efficacy of these systems in evaluating factors mitigating or proliferating disease within respective populations.

6.3 MULTIFACETED EVALUATION OF DISEASE-ASSOCIATED PATHOGENS

There is an inherent range of variability in inferring pathogen presence in Roman Italy with the selected data sources; however, the objective is to systematically identify contextually relevant variables to conceptualize the diverse causal pathways of disease occurrence as a means to target candidate pathogens for further analysis (eg, hybridization capture). Reconstructing the paleoepidemiological context through disease ecology and human–environment interactions using proxy evidence is necessarily limited by the availability of such data and their specificity to the sites studied as well as the degree to which one can infer the potential for pathogen exposure without drawing tenuous interpretations. For example, if parasitic infections are presumed to be part of the disease pool in the Roman Empire, and shotgun sequencing does not detect these pathogens within the coastal and rural skeletal samples within this study, their absence means it is not a focus of further analysis due to a reduced likelihood of success in targeting these pathogens with a molecular capture strategy. The caveat is that although the pathogen is undetected, it does not mean it was not present, thereby requiring cautious interpretation of the metagenomic evidence. Integrating archaeological and literary evidence can facilitate whether these pathogens are suitable for targeting with downstream processing; however, the endeavor is of high risk (diminishing returns). Similarly, the "unexpected" detection of a pathogen is not uncommon, as the historical Greek and Roman literary sources cannot be directly applied to the necropoleis in this study, and archaeological data provide only broad information on the potential (not absolute) hypothesized range of pathogens that may have been present. However, these integrated datasets do provide a framework for hypothesizing the pathogens that may have been present and are practical to pursue in a purposeful manner. The ultimate goal of integrating molecular, archaeological, and literary sources toward a framework of decision-making is to evaluate a variety of separate but interconnected factors that combine to create the ancient disease-scape (Fig. 6.1).

6.4 TOWARD INTERDISCIPLINARY ANCIENT DNA AND PATHOGEN INVESTIGATION STRATEGIES

The perspectives provided by each type of evidence: ancient DNA, written texts, and archaeological data represent one facet of exploring disease in antiquity. Ancient DNA data are a contemporary bio-medical picture of disease, whereas the written and archaeological sources are conceptualizations of a moment in historical time.

The disease ecology at Vagnari, Velia, and Portus Romae is amenable to inferences of factors mitigating or proliferating pathogen exposure, although only a limited range of information is available (eg, climate, extreme weather events) and the resilience of local

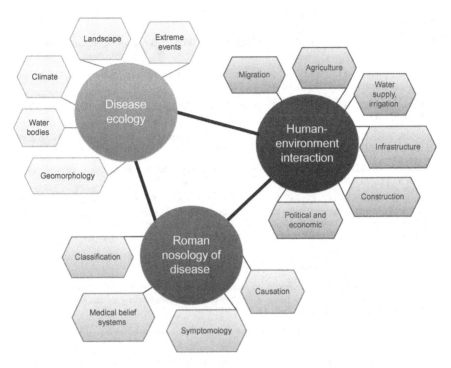

Figure 6.1 Framework integrating aspects of disease ecology, Roman nosology, and the human−environment inter-action to situate molecular data in exploring historical pathogen presence and inferring the experience of disease.

ecosystems to such factors is unknowable. Similarly, humans modify pathways of pathogen exposure by interacting with the environment in diverse ways, whether on the scale of urbanization activities (eg, construction) or day-to-day life (eg, farming, person-to-person contact). Although the context of human activities may be established at the site-level, the consequences of such activities on the long- or short-term composition of the pathogen pool can only be effectively reconstructed by integrating this information with ancient DNA evidence, particularly because skeletal remains often do not display clear evidence of infectious diseases. With metagenomic data, identifying contextually relevant disease-associated pathogens from a sample with high proportions of exogenous DNA presents a formidable, but not insurmountable challenge, requiring a conservative approach toward establishing pathogen presence. It is only through the systematic integration of various evidentiary sources that the complexity of pathogen presence and inferences of the disease experience in the past can begin to be investigated.

REFERENCES

Adams, F., 1891. The Genuine Works of Hippocrates. William Wood and Company, New York, NY.

Adler, C.J., Haak, W., Donlon, D., Cooper, A., 2011. Survival and recovery of DNA from ancient teeth and bone. J. Archaeol. Sci. 38, 956–964.

Aldrete, G., 2007. Floods of the Tiber in Ancient Rome. John Hopkins University Press, Baltimore, MD.

Altschul, S.F., Gish, W., Miller, W., Myers, E.W., Lipman, D.J., 1990. Basic local alignment search tool. J. Mol. Biol. 215, 403–410.

Andersen, J.G., Manchester, K., 1992. The rhinomaxillary syndrome in leprosy: a clinical, radiological, and paleopathological study. Int. J. Osteoarchaeol. 2, 121–129.

Amato, L., Bisogno, G., Cicala, L., Cinque, A., Romano, P., Ruello, M.R., et al., 2010. Palaeo-environmental changes in the archaeological settlement of Elea-Velia: climatic and/or human impact signatures? In: Ciarallo, A., Senatore, M.R. (Eds.), Scienze naturali e archeologia. Il paesaggio antico: interazione uomo/ambiente ed eventi catastrofici. Aracne, Editrice, Rome, pp. 13–16.

Beauchesne, P.D., 2012. Physiological Stress, Bone Growth and Development in Imperial Rome (Unpublished Ph.D. dissertation). University of California, Berkley.

Bellemain, E., Davey, M.L., Kauserud, H., Epp, L.S., Boessenkool, S., Coissac, E., et al., 2013. Fungal palaeodiversity revealed using high-throughput metabarcoding of ancient DNA from arctic permafrost. Environ. Microbiol. 15, 1176–1189.

Bissell, R.A., 1983. Delayed-impact infectious disease after a natural disaster. J. Emerg. Med. 1, 59–66.

Bondioli, L., Macchiarelli, R., Salvadei, L., Passarello, P., 1995. Paleobiologia dell'età romana imperiale: il Progetto "Isola Sacra". In: Peretto, C., Milliken, S. (Eds.), XI Congresso degli Antropologi Italiani. L'Adattamento Umano all'Ambiente. Passato e Presente. Cosmo Iannone Editore, Isernia, pp. 78–79.

Bos, K.I., Schuenemann, V.J., Golding, G.B., Burbano, H.A., Waglechner, N., Coombes, B.K., et al., 2011. A draft genome of Yersinia pestis from victims of the Black Death. Nature 478, 506–510.

Briggs, A.W., Stenzel, U., Meyer, M., Krause, J., Kircher, M., Pääbo, S., 2009. Removal of deaminated cytosines and detection of in vivo methylation in ancient DNA. Nucleic Acids Res. 38 (6), e87.

Brotherton, P., Endicott, P., Sanchez, J.J., Beaumont, M., Barnett, R., Austin, J., et al., 2007. Novel high-resolution characterization of ancient DNA reveals C > U-type base modification events as the sole cause of post mortem miscoding lesions. Nucleic Acids Res. 35, 5717–5728.

Burbano, H.A., Hodges, E., Green, R.E., Briggs, A.W., Krause, J., Meyer, M., et al., 2010. Targeted investigation of the Neandertal genome by array-based sequence capture. Science 328, 723–725.

Carpenter, M.L., Buenrostro, J.D., Valdiosera, C., Schroeder, H., Allentoft, M.E., Sikora, M., et al., 2013. Pulling out the 1%: whole-genome capture for the targeted enrichment of ancient DNA sequencing libraries. Am. J. Hum. Genet. 93, 852–864.

Collier, G.F., 1831. A Translation of the Eight Books of Aul. Corn. Celsus on Medicine. Simpkin and Marshall, London.

Cooper, A., Poinar, H.N., 2000. Ancient DNA: do it right or not at all. Science 289, 1139.

Craig, O.E., Biazzo, M., O'Connell, T.C., Garnsey, P., Martinez-Labarga, C., Lelli, R., et al., 2009. Stable isotopic evidence for diet at the Imperial Roman coastal site of Velia (1st and 2nd Centuries AD) in Southern Italy. Am. J. Phys. Anthropol. 139, 572–583.

Crowe, F., Sperduti, A., O'Connell, T.C., Craig, O.E., Kirsanow, K., Germoni, P., et al., 2010. Water-related occupations and diet in two Roman coastal communities (Italy, first to third century AD): correlation between stable carbon and nitrogen isotope values and auricular exostosis prevalence. Am. J. Phys. Anthropol. 142, 355–366.

Cucina, A., Vargiu, R., Mancinelli, D., Ricci, R., Santandrea, E., Catalano, P., et al., 2006. The necropolis of Vallerano (Rome, 2nd–3rd century AD): an anthropological perspective on the ancient Romans in the Suburbium. Int. J. Osteoarchaeol. 16 (2), 104–117.

Devault, A.M., Golding, B., Waglechner, N., Enk, J.M., Kuch, M., Tien, J.H., et al., 2014a. Second-pandemic strain of *Vibrio cholerae* from the Philadelphia cholera outbreak of 1849. New Engl. J. Med. 370, 334–340.

Devault, A.M., McLoughlin, K., Jaing, C., Gardner, S., Porter, T.M., Enk, J.M., et al., 2014b. Ancient pathogen DNA in archaeological samples detected with a Microbial Detection Array. Sci. Rep. 4, 4245.

Di Rita, F., Celant, A., Magri, D., 2010. Holocene environmental instability in the wetland north of the Tiber delta (Rome, Italy): sea-lake-man interactions. J. Paleolimnol. 44, 51–67.

Drancourt, M., Aboudharam, G., Signoli, M., Dutour, O., Raoult, D., 1998. Detection of 400-year-old *Yersinia pestis* DNA in human dental pulp: an approach to the diagnosis of ancient septicemia. Proc. Natl. Acad. Sci. U.S.A. 95, 12637–12640.

Dyson, S.L., 2010. Rome: A Living Portrait of an Ancient City. John Hopkins University Press, Baltimore, MD.

Eckardt, H., (Ed.), 2010. Roman Diasporas: archaeological approaches to mobility and diversity in the Roman Empire. J. Roman Archaeol., Portsmouth, Suppl. 78, 246.

Facchini, F., Rastelli, E., Brasili, P., 2004. Cribra orbitalia and cribra crania in Roman skeletal remains from the Ravenna area and Rimini (I-IV century AD). Int. J. Osteoarchaeol. 14, 126–136.

Fiammenghi, C.A., 2003. La Necropoli di Elea-Velia: qualche osservazione preliminare. In: Elea-Velia. Le Nuove ricerche. Quaderni del Centro Studi Magna Grecia 1, Naus Editoria, Pozzuoli, Italy, pp. 49–61.

Gilbert, M.T.P., Bandelt, H.J., Hofreiter, M., Barnes, I., 2005. Assessing ancient DNA studies. Trends Ecol. Evol. 20, 541–544.

Ginolhac, A., Rasmussen, M., Gilbert, M.T.P., Willerslev, E., Orlando, L., 2011. mapDamage: testing for damage patterns in ancient DNA sequences. Bioinformatics 27 (15), 2153–2155.

Gowland, R., Garnsey, P., 2010. Skeletal evidence for health, nutritional status and malaria in Rome and the Empire. In: Eckardt, H. (Ed.), Roman Diasporas: Archaeological Approaches to Mobility and Diversity in the Roman Empire. J. Roman Archaeol., Portsmouth, Suppl. 78, pp. 131–156.

Grmek, M.D., 1989. Diseases in the Ancient Greek World (M. Muellner, L. Muellner, Trans.). John Hopkins University Press, Baltimore, MD.

Grove, A.T., Rackham, O., 2001. The Nature of Mediterranean Europe: An Ecological History. Yale University Press, New Haven, CT.

Higgins, D., Austin, J.J., 2013. Teeth as a source of DNA for forensic identification of human remains: a review. Sci. Justice 53, 433–441.

Hofreiter, M., Paijmans, J.L.A., Goodchild, H., Speller, C.F., Barlow, A., Fortes, G.G., et al., 2014. The future of ancient DNA: technical advances and conceptual shifts. Bioessays 37, 284–293.

Huson, D.H., Auch, A.F., Qi, J., Schuster, S.C., 2007. MEGAN analysis of metagenomic data. Genome Res. 17 (3), 377–386.

Ivers, L.C., Ryan, E.T., 2006. Infectious diseases of severe weather-related and flood-related natural disasters. Curr. Opin. Infect. Dis. 19, 408–414.

Jouanna, J., 1999. Hippocrates. (M.B. DeBevoise, Trans.). John Hopkins University Press, Baltimore.

Kay, G.L., Sergeant, M.J., Giuffra, V., Bandiera, P., Milanese, M., Bramanti, B., et al., 2014. Recovery of a medieval *Brucella melitensis* genome using shotgun metagenomics. MBio 5 (4), e01337-14.

Keay, S.J., Paroli, L. (Eds.), 2011. Portus and Its Hinterland: Recent Archaeological Research, vol. 18. British School at Rome, London, Archaeological Monographs of the British School at Rome, London.

Keiser, J., de Castro, M.C., Maltese, M.F., Bos, R., Tanner, M., Singer, B.H., et al., 2005. Effect of irrigation and large dams on the burden of malaria on a global and regional scale. Am. J. Trop. Med. Hyg. 72 (4), 392–406.

Killgrove, K., 2010. Migration and Mobility in Imperial Rome (Unpublished Ph.D. dissertation). University of North Carolina at Chapel Hill, Chapel Hill.

Killgrove, K., 2014. Bioarchaeology in the Roman Empire. Encyclopedia of Global Archaeology. Springer, New York, NY, pp. 876–882.

Kircher, M., Sawyer, S., Meyer, M., 2012. Double indexing overcomes inaccuracies in multiplex sequencing on the Illumina platform. Nucleic Acids Res. 40, e3.

Krieger, N., 2008. Proximal, distal, and the politics of causation: what's level got to do with it? Am. J. Public Health 98, 221–230.

Krieger, N., 2011. Epidemiology and the People's Health: Theory and Context. Oxford University Press, Oxford.

Kühn, C.G. (Ed.), 1825. Claudii Galeni Opera Omnia, 20 vols. Georg Olms Verlag, Hildesheim, Reprint.

Legendre, M., Bartoli, J., Shmakova, L., Jeudy, S., Labadie, K., Adrait, A., et al., 2014. Thirty-thousand-year-old distant relative of giant icosahedral DNA viruses with a pandoravirus morphology. Proc. Natl. Acad. Sci. U.S.A. 111, 4274–4279.

Leven, K.H., 2004. "At times these ancient facts seem to lie before me like a patient on a hospital bed"—retrospective diagnosis and ancient medical history. In: Horstmanshoff, H.F.J., Stol, M., van Tilburg, C.R. (Eds.), Magic and Rationality in Ancient Near Eastern and Graeco-Roman Medicine. Brill Academic Publishers, Boston, MA, pp. 369–386.

Lindahl, T., 1993. Instability and decay of the primary structure of DNA. Nature 362, 709–715.

Meyer, M., Kircher, M., 2010. Illumina sequencing library preparation for highly multiplexed target capture and sequencing. Cold Spring Harb. Protoc. 2010 (6), pdb.prot5448.

Mitchell, P.D., 2011. Retrospective diagnosis and the use of historical texts for investigating disease in the past. Int. J. Palaeopathol. 1, 81–88.

Molak, M., Ho, S.Y.W., 2011. Evaluating the impact of post-mortem damage in ancient DNA: a theoretical approach. J. Mol. Evol. 73, 244–255.

Muramoto, O., 2014. Retrospective diagnosis of a famous historical figure: ontological, epistemic, and ethical considerations. Philos. Ethics Humanit. Med. 9, 10.

Nutton, V., 2004. Ancient Medicine. Routledge, London.

Orlando, L., Gilbert, M.T.P., Willerslev, E., 2015. Reconstructing ancient genomes and epigenomes. Nat. Rev. Genet. 6, 395–408.

Ortner, D.J., 2008. Differential diagnosis of skeletal lesions in infectious disease. In: Pinhasi, R., Mays, S. (Eds.), Advances in Human Palaeopathology. John Wiley & Sons Ltd, Chichester, pp. 191–214.

Pääbo, S., Poinar, H.N., Serre, D., Jaenicke-Despres, V., Hebler, J., Rohland, N., et al., 2004. Genetic analyses from ancient DNA. Annu. Rev. Genet. 38, 645–679.

Page, D.L., 1953. Thucydides description of the great plague at Athens. Classical Quart. 3 (3–4), 97–119.

Prowse, T.L., Schwarcz, H.P., Saunders, S.R., Macchiarelli, R., Bondioli, L., 2005. Isotopic evidence for age-related variation in diet from Isola Sacra, Italy. Am. J. Phys. Anthropol. 128, 2–13.

Prowse, T.L., Schwarcz, H.P., Garnsey, P., Knyf, M., Macchiarelli, R., Bondioli, L., 2007. Isotopic evidence for age-related immigration to imperial Rome. Am. J. Phys. Anthropol. 132, 510–519.

Prowse, T., Barta, J.L., von Hunnius, T.E., Small, A.M., 2010. Stable isotope and mtDNA evidence for geographic origins at the site of Vagnari, south Italy. In: Eckardt, H. (Ed.), Roman Diasporas: Archaeological Approaches to Mobility and Diversity in the Roman Empire. J. Roman Archaeol., Portsmouth, Suppl. 78, pp. 175–198.

Prowse, T.L., Nause, C., Ledger, M., 2014. Growing up and growing old on an imperial estate: preliminary palaeopathological analysis of skeletal remains from Vagnari. In: Small, A.M. (Ed.), Beyond Vagnari. Edipuglia, Bari, pp. 111–122.

Rackham, H., 1938. Natural History by Pliny the Elder. (H. Rackham Trans.). W. Heinemann, London.

Roberts, C., Manchester, K., 2005. The Archaeology of Disease, third ed. Cornell University Press, Ithaca, NY.

Rosenberg, C.E., 1992. Framing disease: illness, society and history. In: Rosenberg, C.E., Golden, J. (Eds.), Framing Disease: Studies in Cultural History. Rutgers University Press, New Jersey, pp. iii–xxvi.

Ruello, M.R., 2008. Geoarchaeology in Coastal Areas of Campania: The Sites of Neapolis and Elea—Velia (Unpublished Ph.D. dissertation). University of Naples Federico II, Italy.

Sadori, L., Jahns, S., Peyron, O., 2011. Mid-Holocene vegetation history of the central Mediterranean. Holocene 21, 117–129.

Sallares, R., 2002. Malaria and Rome: A History of Malaria in Ancient Italy. Oxford University Press, Oxford.

Scheidel, W., 2003. Germs for Rome. In: Edwards, C., Woolf, G. (Eds.), Rome the Cosmopolis. Cambridge University Press, Cambridge, pp. 158–176.

Scheidel, W., 2009. Disease and death in the ancient city of Rome. Princeton/Stanford Working Papers in Classics. Stanford University.

Schwarz, C., Debruyne, R., Kuch, M., McNally, E., Schwarcz, H., Aubrey, A.D., et al., 2009. New insights from old bones: DNA preservation and degradation in permafrost preserved mammoth remains. Nucleic Acids Res. 37, 3215–3229.

Scobie, A., 1986. Slums, sanitation, and mortality in the Roman world. Klio 68, 399–433.

Skoglund, P., Northoff, B.H., Shunkov, M.V., Derevianko, A.P., Paabo, S., Krause, J., et al., 2014. Separating endogenous ancient DNA from modern day contamination in a Siberian Neandertal. Proc. Natl. Acad. Sci. U.S.A. 111, 2229–2234.

Small, A.M. (Ed.), 2011. Vagnari. The Village, the Industries the Imperial Property. Edipuglia, Bari.

Small, A.M. (Ed.), 2014. Beyond Vagnari: New Themes in the Study of Roman South Italy. Edipuglia, Bari.

Spigelman, M., Donoghue, H.D., Abdeen, Z., Ereqat, S., Sarie, I., Greenblatt, C.L., et al., 2015. Evolutionary changes in the genome of *Mycobacterium tuberculosis* and the human genome from 9000 years BP until modern times. Tuberculosis 95, S145–S149.

St. John, J., 2011. SeqPrep. < https://github.com/jstjohn/SeqPrep > (accessed 02.05.15).

Steinbock, R.T., 1976. Paleopathological Diagnosis and Interpretation: Bone Diseases in Ancient Human Populations. Charles C. Thomas, Springfield.

Sutherst, R.W., 2004. Global change and human vulnerability to vector-borne diseases. Clin. Microbiol. Rev. 17 (1), 136–173.

Wagner, D.M., Klunk, J., Harbeck, M., Devault, A., Waglechner, N., Sahl, J.W., et al., 2014. Yersinia pestis and the plague of Justinian 541-543 AD: a genomic analysis. Lancet Infect. Dis. 14, 319–326.

Waltner-Toews, D., 2001. An ecosystem approach to health and its applications to tropical and emerging diseases. Reports Public Health 17, 7–36.

Warinner, C., Speller, C., Collins, M.J., 2015. A new era in palaeomicrobiology: prospects for ancient dental calculus as a long-term record of the human oral microbiome. Philos. Trans. R. Soc. Lond. B 370 (1660), 20130376.

Whatmore, A.M., 2014. Ancient-pathogen genomics: coming of age? mBio 5, e01676-14.

World Health Organization, 2015. About vector-borne diseases. <http://www.who.int/campaigns/world-health-day/2014/vector-borne-diseases/en/> (accessed 03.02.16.).

Wood, J.W., Milner, G.R., Harpending, H.C., Weiss, K.M., 1992. The osteological paradox: problems of inferring prehistoric health from skeletal samples. Curr. Anthropol. 33, 343–370.

Wright, L.E., Yoder, C.J., 2003. Recent progress in bioarchaeology: approaches to the osteological paradox. J. Archaeol. Res 11 (1), 43–70.

Yasuoka, J., Levins, R., 2007. Impact of deforestation and agricultural development on Anopheline ecology and malaria epidemiology. Am. J. Trop. Med. Hyg. 76 (3), 450–460.

CHAPTER 7

The Use of Linguistic Data in Bioarchaeological Research: An Example From the American Southwest

M.A. Schillaci[1] and S. Wichmann[2,3]

[1]Department of Anthropology, University of Toronto Scarborough, Toronto, ON, Canada
[2]Leiden University Centre for Linguistics, Leiden University, Leiden, The Netherlands
[3]Laboratory of Quantitative Linguistics, Kazan Federal University, Kazan, Russia

7.1 INTRODUCTION

It has been suggested that the genes, language, and culture of ethnic groups in the prehistoric American Southwest need not have evolved together as a package in bounded social groups (Ortman, 2012). Consequently, genetic, linguistic, and cultural heritage may not have followed parallel patterns of descent (Ortman, 2012). To address this question of coevolution, a greater understanding of the relationship among datasets describing genetic, linguistic, and cultural variation for the archaeological groups of interest is needed. In this chapter we explore this notion of coevolution by examining the correlation of linguistic and genetic relationships among ancestral and present-day Tanoan-speaking Pueblo Indians of northern New Mexico. In addition, we examine the effects of geographic distance on linguistic and biological relationships by formally testing an isolation-by-distance model.

7.1.1 Previous Research

The Tanoan languages, Tiwa, Tewa, and Towa, along with Kiowa, belong to the Kiowa-Tanoan language family. Tiwa and Tewa are spoken at various pueblos within the Rio Grande Valley of north-central New Mexico, while Towa is spoken at Jemez Pueblo located on the banks of the Jemez River west of the Rio Grande Valley (Fig. 7.1). Although the languages, culture, archaeology, and biological variation of the Tanoan-speaking Pueblo Indians have received considerable

Beyond the Bones. DOI: http://dx.doi.org/10.1016/B978-0-12-804601-2.00007-7

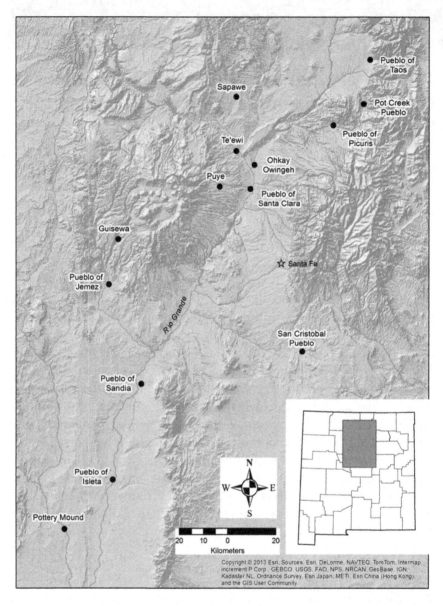

Figure 7.1 Map showing pueblo locations within the Rio Grande Valley of New Mexico. Map generated using ArcGIS.

attention in the anthropological literature (see Ortman, 2012, for a review), very little research has examined the relationships among these disparate datasets in a formal way. In their study of the population history and social organization of prehistoric Tewa, Schillaci and Stojanowski (2005) examined the effect of geographic distance on the genetic relationships among ancestral Tewa pueblos (c. AD 1350–1680), estimated using craniometric data. The results of the Mantel tests employed in that study indicated only a weak and statistically nonsignificant correlation ($r = 0.443$, $p = 0.261$) between geographic and genetic distances, suggesting that geography was not the primary basis of gene flow. Although not focused on Tanoan-speaking populations, research by Kemp et al. (2010) utilizing Mantel tests, found significant partial correlations (controlling for correlation with geographic distance) between genetic distances based on Y-chromosome variation and linguistic distances ($r = 0.33–0.384$; $p < 0.02$) among populations from the American Southwest and Mesoamerica, including the Tanoan-speaking population from Jemez Pueblo. The partial correlations between genetic distances based on mitochondrial DNA (mtDNA) and linguistic distances were not significant ($r = 0.124–0.153$; $p > 0.05$). Partial correlations (controlling for either Y-chromosome variation or mtDNA variation) between geographic distances and linguistic distances were low, ranging from between $r = 0.321$ and $r = 0.153$, and mostly nonsignificant ($p = 0.033–0.196$).

More recently, Ortman (2012) examined linguistic and craniometric datasets, as well as oral tradition and estimates of population size based on room counts at habitation sites in his analysis of Tewa ancestry. After careful evaluation of the results from the various analyses of these data, Ortman proposed that the ancestral Tewa people and language were brought to the northern Rio Grande Valley from the Mesa Verde region of southwestern Colorado by way of a large population movement. Although Ortman's study—by far, the most comprehensive to date—utilized disparate datasets, he did not incorporate multiple datasets into a formal analytical model. Here, we examine the correlation between language and genetic relationships among extant and ancestral Tanoan pueblos, and the effect of geographic distance on those relationships, using a formal analytical model.

7.2 METHODS

In order to estimate the relationships among Tanoan languages we generated pair-wise measures of lexical dissimilarity based on a 40-word subset (Table 7.1) of the Swadesh 100-word list using the Automated Similarity Judgment Program (Holman et al., 2011).

Table 7.1 40-Word Subset of the Swadesh 100-Word List (Swadesh, 1955) Used by the ASJP to Generate the LDND Measures of Lexical Dissimilarity Among Languages

Swadesh No.	Word	Swadesh No.	Word
1	I	47	Knee
2	You	48	Hand
3	We	51	Breast
11	One	53	Liver
12	Two	54	Drink
18	Person	57	See
19	Fish	58	Hear
21	Dog	61	Die
22	Louse	66	Come
23	Tree	72	Sun
25	Leaf	74	Star
28	Skin	75	Water
30	Blood	77	Stone
31	Bone	82	Fire
34	Horn	85	Path
39	Ear	86	Mountain
40	Eye	92	Night
41	Nose	95	Full
43	Tooth	96	New
44	Tongue	100	Name

This list of 40 words has been found to yield lexicostatistical results at least as accurate as the full 100-word list as determined by their correlation with language classifications by specialists (Holman et al., 2008). Using the shorter list allowed us to obtain complete datasets for all Kiowa-Tanoan languages. Tanoan words were gathered from the literature, experts, and native speakers by L. Sutton. Sources for the word lists are as follows. Southern Tewa (Arizona Tewa): Kroskrity (1993), Kroskrity and Healing (1978, 1980), Yegerlehner (1957); Rio Grande Tewa, including the San Juan and Santa Clara dialects: Kroskrity (1993), Harrington (1916), Hale (1967), Dozier (1953), Hoijer and Dozier (1949), Martinez (1982), Speirs (1966), Speirs and Speirs (1979), Wycliffe Bible Translators (1969); Towa (or Jemez): Hale (1967), Gatschet (1876), Yumitani (1998); Hale (1956–1957); Northern Tiwa (Taos Pueblo): Hale (1967), Trager and Trager (1959),

Yu (2006), Harrington (1910), Trager (1935–1972), Trager (1946); Southern Tiwa (Sandia and Isleta Pueblos): Frantz (n.d.), Gatschet (1879), Leap (1970), and the Wycliffe Bible Translators (1978). For this analysis, Arizona Tewa is assumed to represent Southern Tewa (Tano). This assumption is commonly, though not universally (see Ortman, 2012), accepted. The dialect spoken at Taos was used to represent Northern Tiwa.

We used a measure of lexical dissimilarity based on a Levenshtein distance (LD), which is defined as the minimum number of successive changes needed to change one word to another, where each change is either a deletion, insertion, or substitution of a symbol representing a class of speech sounds (Holman et al., 2011, p. 843). The resulting value is then normalized by dividing the LD by the number of symbols of the longer of the two words. This results in a normalized Levenshtein distance (LDN) that corrects for differences in word length. A LDN divided (LDND) is then calculated by dividing the average LDN for all the word pairs involving the same meaning by the average LDN for all pairs of words referring to different concepts (Holman et al., 2011, p. 843). The LDN in the denominator, then, is the mean of $(40 \times 39)/2$ off-diagonal comparisons in a 40-by-40 item matrix of concepts. This normalization penalizes the overall similarity when words not referring to the same concepts are accidentally similar, thus correcting for chance similarity due to similar sound inventories. In the special case where words with different meanings are on average more similar than words with the same meanings, a LDND of greater than 100% will be the outcome. Using LDND rather than LDN has been shown to lead to more accurate classification results (Wichmann et al., 2010).

To estimate genetic relationships we calculated biological distances derived from the genetic relationship, or R-matrix (Relethford and Blangero, 1990; Relethford et al., 1997), based on craniometric data using Dr J. Relethford's RMET 5.0 software program (see http://employees.oneonta.edu/relethjh/programs/). The craniometric data for 12 variables (Table 7.2) were obtained from skeletal populations known to be directly ancestral to the same pueblos from which the linguistic data were derived (Table 7.3), with the possible exception of Pottery Mound, which may have included non-Tiwa immigrants from the west (Eckert, 2008). These data were generously provided

Table 7.2 Craniometric Variables Used in the Analysis

Variable	Abbreviation	Measurements[a]
Upper facial height	NPH	Nasion-prosthion
Upper facial breadth	UFB	Frontomalare—frontomalare
Minimum frontal breadth	WFB	Frontotemporale—frontotemporale
Bizygomatic breadth	ZYB	Zygion—zygion
Orbital breadth	OBB	Dacryon—ectoconchion
Orbital height	OBH	Perpendicular to OBB at midpoint
Interorbital breadth	DKB	Dacryon—dacryon
Biorbital breadth	EKB	Ectoconchion—ectoconchion
Nasal height	NLH	Nasion—nasospinale
Nasal breadth	NLB	Alare—alare
Palate length	MAL	Prosthion—alveolon
Palate breadth	MAB	Ectomalare—ectomalare

[a]See Howells (1973) and Steele and Bramblett (1988) for definition of cranial landmarks and measurements.

Table 7.3 Information on the Tanoan Populations Included in the Analysis

Pueblo	n	Language	Time Period
San Juan (OhkayOwingeh)		Tewa	Historic—Present
Santa Clara		Tewa	Historic—Present
Jemez		Towa	Historic—Present
Sandia		Southern Tiwa	Historic—Present
Isleta		Southern Tiwa	Historic—Present
Taos		Northern Tiwa	AD 1450—Present
Picuris	7	Northern Tiwa	AD 1200?—Present
Pot Creek	10	Northern Tiwa	AD 1250—1320
Sapawe	17	San Juan Tewa	AD 1350—1525
Te'ewi	9	San Juan Tewa	AD 1250—1500
Puye	58	Santa Clara Tewa	AD 1325—1540
San Cristobal	41	Southern Tewa	AD 1325—1675
Guisewa	7	Towa	AD 1400—1540
Amoxiumqua	7	Towa	AD 1325—1540
Kwasteyukwa	28	Towa	AD 1400—1540
Pottery Mound	27	Southern Tiwa	AD 1300—1500

n denotes sample sizes for the ancestral skeletal populations from which craniometric data were collected. See Fig. 7.1 for locations.

by S. Ortman, and are the same used in his recent study of Tewa ancestry (Ortman, 2012). To increase sample sizes the male and female data were pooled after conducting within-sex z-score transformations. These transformed data were then pooled by language grouping before calculating biological distances. We generated neighbor-joining trees (Saitou and Nei, 1987) based on the linguistic and biological distance matrices using MEGA 6.0 (Tamura et al., 2013). These trees describe the historical or evolutionary relationships among either the Tanoan languages or populations (pueblos) included in our study.

Geographic (straight-line) distances (km) among pueblos were measured using the ruler tool with mouse navigation in Google Earth. We use the measured geographic distance among pueblos to test a generalized isolation-by-distance model borrowed from the field of population genetics (Wright, 1943). This model predicts that divergence among populations will be proportional to geographic distances due to the isolating effects of spatial separation on the magnitude of genetic or linguistic exchange such as borrowing. For our analytical model we used distance matrix correlation analyses (Mantel tests) to examine the relationship between linguistic and biological distance matrices, and to test a generalized isolation-by-distance model. The Mantel tests were conducted using MANTEL 3.1 (see http://employees.oneonta.edu/relethjh/programs/).

7.3 RESULTS

The lexical and biological distances are presented in Table 7.4. The structure of relationships among Tanoan languages described

Table 7.4 Lexical (LDND) and Biological (R-Matrix)[a] Distances Among Language Groupings

	SJT	STE	TOW	STI	SCT	NTI
1. San Juan Tewa (SJT)	0.00	0.041	0.016	0.111	0.036	0.093
2. Southern Tewa (STE)	29.09	0.00	0.026	0.098	0.029	0.011
3. Towa (TOW)	86.46	90.22	0.00	0.201	0.036	0.102
4. Southern Tiwa (STI)	76.94	82.97	89.03	0.00	0.138	0.076
5. Santa Clara Tewa (SCT)	11.14	36.44	86.74	76.46	0.00	0.054
6. Northern Tiwa (NTI)	76.76	79.07	89.32	45.90	77.61	0.00

Lexical distances are listed below the shaded diagonal, with biological distances listed above the diagonal.
[a]*R-matrix distances were calculated using a narrow-sense heritability $h^2 = 0.55$ with relative population weights set to 1.*

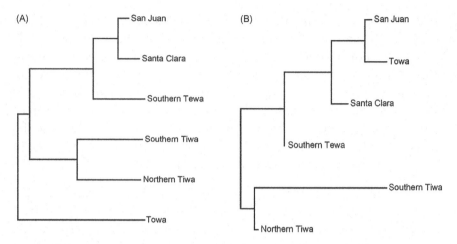

Figure 7.2 Neighbor-joining trees based on (A) linguistic distances, and (B) biological distances.

by the neighbor-joining tree derived from the lexical data (Fig. 7.2A) is consistent with what has been presented by Davis (1959) based on shared cognates, and with that presented by Ortman (2012) based on shared phonetic innovations. As expected, Towa appears as the sister to two separate clades comprising the Tewa and Tiwa language dialects respectively. The tree describing the biological relationships among populations (Fig. 7.2B) is visibly similar to the lexical tree, with the exception of the Towa population, which is placed within the Tewa grouping, or clade. As was seen in the tree based on lexical data, the two Tiwa populations again form a single clade. The appearance of a Tiwa clade and a largely Tewa clade suggests that there may be some degree of linguistic structuring to biological relationships. Interestingly, the population from Pottery Mound appears to be closely related biologically to the Northern Tiwa population from Pot Creek and Picuris, suggesting this pueblo is likely made up primarily of Southern Tiwa residents rather than non-Tiwa immigrants.

Although the trees describing linguistic and biological relationships exhibited moderately similar structure visually, the results of the Mantel test indicate that there is not a significant relationship between linguistic and biological distances ($r = 0.309$, $p = 0.171$). It is important to note, however, that the linguistic distances were generated from data collected during the 19th and 20th centuries, and therefore partly reflect linguistic change that has occurred after the occupation of the pueblos from which the craniometric data were derived. In other words, the linguistic variation analyzed in our study has been subject to the historical and evolutionary processes that influence the relationships among populations for a longer period of time. Although this time difference between datasets may have reduced to some degree the correlation between linguistic and biological relationships, its effect was likely not great. The isolation-by-distance model was rejected for both language ($r = 0.520$, $p = 0.068$) and biological relationships ($r = 0.305$, $p = 0.094$), suggesting that linguistic and biological differences are not mediated by geographic proximity, at least not in this case and at this level of resolution.

7.4 DISCUSSION AND CONCLUSIONS

The present study illustrates the potential utility of linguistic data in bioarchaeological analyses of population history. Our results support the suggestion that genes and languages have not evolved together as a package among Tanoan pueblos (cf. Ortman, 2012). In other words, the genetic and linguistic heritage of Tanoans may not have followed parallel patterns of descent. Furthermore, linguistic and biological relationships among pueblos do not seem to have been mediated primarily by geographic proximity. Our results suggest that gene flow across linguistic boundaries was likely common. In particular, gene flow with the Towa speaking pueblo of Jemez seems to have been pronounced among Tewa pueblos, despite greater linguistic and geographic distances. This would be consistent with the suggestion by Schillaci and Stojanowski (2005) that gene flow among ancestral pueblos may have been mediated through a complex social network built on reciprocal exchange of esoteric knowledge and ritual paraphernalia (see Ware and Blinman, 1998), given that exchange within such a network need not be proportional to geographic proximity. While intriguing, there is no way to test whether or not a ritual exchange network existed, and if it did, whether or not it mediated linguistic and genetic exchange. There are myriad factors other than isolation by geographic distance that could have shaped the linguistic, genetic, and cultural variation among Tanoan pueblos, including ancestry, migration, and the historical and economic processes associated with subsistence, population aggregation and integration, and the control and exchange of raw materials (cf. Wendorf and Reed, 1955; McNutt, 1969; Ford et al., 1972; Fowles, 2004a,b; Fowles et al., 2007; Boyer et al., 2010; Ortman, 2012). Future holistic integrative research on Tanoan prehistory should incorporate the disparate datasets reflecting such processes. Importantly, future research should also utilize quantitative analyses that incorporate such disparate datasets in a formal analytical framework.

ACKNOWLEDGMENTS

We are grateful to the following individuals who contributed to this research. Logan Sutton compiled and edited the word lists used in this study, expanding on the existing Automated Similarity Judgment Program database (Wichmann et al., 2013). The added lexical data were transcribed by Julia Bischoffberger. This paper benefited greatly from discussions with S. Lakatos and S. Ortman. We would like to thank the editors Madeleine Mant and Alyson Holland for inviting us to contribute to this volume. MAS's research was funded in part by a grant from the Social Sciences and Research Council (SSHRC) of Canada. SW's research was funded by the ERC Advanced Grant MesAndLin(g)k, Proj. No. 295918, and by a subsidy from the Russian Government to support the Program of Competitive Development of Kazan Federal University.

REFERENCES

Boyer, J.L., Moore, J.L., Lakatos, S.A., Akins, N.J., Wilson, C.D., Blinman, E., 2010. Remodeling immigration: a northern Rio Grande perspective on depopulation, migration, and donation-side models. In: Kohler, T.A., Varien, M.D., Wright, A. (Eds.), Leaving Mesa Verde: Peril and Change in the Thirteenth-Century Southwest. University of Arizona Press, Tucson, AZ, pp. 285–323.

Davis, I., 1959. Linguistic clues to northern Rio Grande prehistory. El Palacio 66, 73–84.

Dozier, E.P., 1953. Tewa II: verb structure. Int. J. Am. Linguist. 19, 118–127.

Eckert, S.L., 2008. Pottery and Practice: The Expression of Identity at Pottery Mound and Hummingbird Pueblo. University of New Mexico Press, Albuquerque, NM.

Ford, R.I., Schroeder, A.H., Peckham, S.L., 1972. Three perspectives on Puebloan prehistory. In: Ortiz, A. (Ed.), New Perspectives on the Pueblos. University of New Mexico Press, Albuquerque, NM, pp. 19–30.

Fowles, S.M., 2004a. The Making of Made People: The Prehistoric Evolution of Hierocracy Among the Northern Tiwa of New Mexico (unpublished PhD thesis). University of Michigan, Ann Arbor, MI.

Fowles, S.M., 2004b. Tewa versus Tiwa. In: Adams, E.C., Duff, A.I. (Eds.), The Protohistoric Pueblo World AD 1275-1600. University of Arizona Press, Tucson, pp. 17–25.

Fowles, S.M., Minc, L., Duwe, S., Hill, D.V., 2007. Clay, conflict, and village aggregation: compositional analyses of pre-Classic pottery from Taos, New Mexico. Am. Antiquity 72, 125–152.

Frantz, D., n.d. Lexicon of Isleta Tiwa (unpublished manuscript).

Gatschet, A.S., 1876. Zwölf Sprachen aus dem Südwesten Amerikas. Hermann Böhlau, Weimar.

Gatschet, A.S., 1879. Classification into seven linguistic stocks of Western Indian dialects contained in forty vocabularies. In: Wheeler, G.M. (Ed.), Report on United States Geographical Surveys West of the One Hundredth Meridian, vol. 7, Archaeology, Appendix, Linguistics. Government Printing Office, Washington, DC, pp. 403–485.

Hale, K.L., 1956–1957. Unpublished notes on Jemez grammar.

Hale, K.L., 1967. Toward a reconstruction of Kiowa-Tanoan phonology. Int. J. Am. Linguist. 33, 112–120.

Harrington, J.P., 1910. An introductory paper on the Tiwa language, dialect of Taos, New Mexico. Am. Anthropol. 12, 11–48.

Harrington, J.P., 1916. The ethnogeography of the Tewa Indians. 29th Annual Report of the Bureau of American Ethnology. Government Printing Office, Washington, DC.

Hoijer, H., Dozier, E.P., 1949. The phonemes of Tewa, Santa Clara dialect. Int. J. Am. Linguist. 15, 139–144.

Holman, E.W., Wichmann, S., Brown, C.H., Velupillai, V., Müller, A., Brown, P., et al., 2008. Explorations in automated language classification. Folia Linguist. 42, 331–354.

Holman, E.W., Brown, C.H., Wichmann, S., Müller, A., Velupillai, V., Hammarström, H., et al., 2011. Automated dating of the world's language families based on lexical similarity. Curr. Anthropol. 52, 841–875.

Howells, W.W., 1973. Cranial variation in man. A study by multivariate analysis of patterns of difference among recent human populations. Pap. Peabody. Mus. Am. A 67, 1–259.

Kemp, B.M., González-Oliver, A., Malhi, R.S., Monroe, C., Schroeder, K.B., McDonough, J., et al., 2010. Evaluating the farming/language dispersal hypothesis with genetic variation exhibited by populations in the Southwest and Mesoamerica. Proc. Natl. Acad. Sci. USA 107, 6759–6764.

Kroskrity, P.V., 1993. Language, History, and Identity: Ethnolinguistic Studies of the Arizona Tewa. University of Arizona Press, Tucson, AZ.

Kroskrity, P.V., Healing, D., 1978. Coyote and bullsnake. In: Bright, W. (Ed.), Coyote Stories I IJAL Native American Texts Series, Monograph 1. University of Chicago Press, Chicago, IL, pp. 162–170.

Kroskrity, P.V., Healing, D., 1980. Coyote woman and the deer children. In: Kendall, M.B. (Ed.), Coyote Stories II. IJAL Native American Texts Series, Monograph 6. University of Chicago Press, Chicago, pp. 119–128.

Leap, W.L., 1970. The Language of Isleta, New Mexico (unpublished PhD thesis). Southern Methodist University, Dallas.

Martinez, E., 1982. San Juan Pueblo Téwa Dictionary. Bishop Publishing, Portales.

McNutt, C.H., 1969. Early Puebloan occupations at Tesuque by-pass and the upper Rio Grande Valley. Anthropological Papers No. 40. Museum of Anthropology. University of Michigan, Ann Arbor, MI.

Ortman, S.G., 2012. Winds from the North: Tewa Origins and Historical Anthropology. University of Utah Press, Salt Lake City, UT.

Relethford, J.H., Blangero, J., 1990. Detection of differential gene flow from patterns of quantitative variation. Hum. Biol. 63, 629–641.

Relethford, J.H., Crawford, M.H., Blangero, J., 1997. Genetic drift and gene flow in post-famine Ireland. Hum. Biol. 69, 443–465.

Saitou, N., Nei, M., 1987. The neighbor-joining method: a new method for reconstructing phylogenetic trees. Mol. Biol. Evol. 4, 406–425.

Schillaci, M.A., Stojanowski, C.M., 2005. Craniometric variation and the population history of the prehistoric Tewa. Am. J. Phys. Anthropol. 126, 404–412.

Speirs, R.H., 1966. Some aspects of the structure of Rio Grande Tewa (unpublished PhD thesis). State University of New York Buffalo, Buffalo.

Speirs, R.H., Speirs, A., 1979. Tewa Workbook. Summer Institute of Linguistics, Huntington Beach, CA.

Steele, D.G., Bramblett, C.A., 1988. The Anatomy and Biology of the Human Skeleton. Texas A&M Press, College Station, TX.

Swadesh, M., 1955. Towards greater accuracy in lexicostatistical dating. Int. J. Am. Linguist. 21, 121–137.

Tamura, K., Stecher, G., Peterson, D., Filipski, A., Kumar, S., 2013. MEGA6: molecular evolutionary genetics analysis version 6.0. Mol. Biol. Evol. 30, 2725–2729.

Trager, G.L., 1935–1972. The Papers of George L. Trager. University of California-Irvine, Langson Library Special Collections and Archives, unpublished notes.

Trager, G.L., 1946. An outline of Taos grammar. In: Osgood, C. (Ed.), Linguistic Structures of Native America. Viking Fund, New York, NY, pp. 184–221.

Trager, G.L., Trager, E.C., 1959. Kiowa and Tanoan. Am. Anthropol. 61, 1078–1083.

Ware, J.A., Blinman, E., 1998. Cultural collapse and reorganization: the origin and spread of Pueblo ritual sodalities. In: Hegmon, M. (Ed.), The Archaeology of Regional Interaction in the Prehistoric Southwest. University of Colorado Press, Boulder, CO, pp. 381–409.

Wendorf, F., Reed, E.K., 1955. An alternative reconstruction of northern Rio Grande prehistory. El Palacio 62, 131–173.

Wichmann, S., Holman, E.W., Bakker, D., Brown, C.H., 2010. Evaluating linguistic distance measures. Physica A 389, 3632–3639.

Wichmann, S., Müller, A., Wett, A., Velupillai, V., Bischoffberger, J., Brown, C.H., et al., 2013. The ASJP Database (version 16). <http://asjp.clld.org/> (accessed 20.01.16).

Wright, S., 1943. Isolation by distance. Genetics 28, 114–138.

Wycliffe Bible Translators, 1969. Mark itaʾnannin: Jesus Christ-víʾgedi.

Wycliffe Bible Translators, 1978. Mark nashiamiwe Jesus Christ-ʿayti. Selected portions from Mark in the Tiwa language of Isleta Pueblo. (B. Allen, D. Gardiner, Trans.).

Yegerlehner, J.F., 1957. Phonology and Morphology of Hopi-Tewa (unpublished PhD thesis). Indiana University, Bloomington, IN.

Yu, D., 2006. Comparative phonology of Picurís and Taos. Available from: <http://linguistics. berkeley.edu/~dom/historical-picuris.pdf> (accessed 2.01.16).

Yumitani, Y., 1998. A Phonology and Morphology of Jemez Towa (unpublished PhD thesis). University of Kansas, Laurence, KS.

CHAPTER 8

The Present Informs the Past: Incorporating Modern Clinical Data Into Paleopathological Analyses of Metabolic Bone Disease

L. Lockau

Department of Anthropology, McMaster University, Hamilton, ON, Canada

8.1 INTRODUCTION

Paleopathology, the study of disease in antiquity (Ortner, 2011), exists at the intersection of medicine and anthropology (Cook and Powell, 2006). The unique integration of these two disciplines, through contextualization of clinical data using anthropological perspectives, forms the basis of paleopathological understandings of health in the past. However, clinical sciences and anthropology are sometimes characterized as contrasting rather than collaborating forces (Armelagos, 2003; Buikstra, 2010; Bush and Zvelebil, 1991; Meiklejohn and Zvelebil, 1991; Zuckerman and Armelagos, 2011). While perceived dichotomies between method and theory, biology and culture, description and interpretation, and process and categorization often serve to reinforce contrast and tension (Armelagos and Van Gerven, 2003; Huss-Ashmore et al., 1982; Washburn, 1951), it is productive to reconceptualize this relationship as integrative by recognizing that the value of a multifaceted analysis is greater than the sum of its parts. This paper will examine ways in which paleopathological analyses of skeletal evidence for metabolic bone disease have applied clinical data, as well as limitations associated with using clinical information in this context. Uses of clinical data reveal attitudes toward the relative value of clinical approaches to and understandings of metabolic bone disease for methodological, interpretive, and theoretical aspects of paleopathological analysis.

The term metabolic bone disease can refer to any condition that interferes with normal skeletal metabolism, by disrupting normal

Beyond the Bones. DOI: http://dx.doi.org/10.1016/B978-0-12-804601-2.00008-9

bone formation, mineralization, remodeling, or a combination of these processes (Brickley and Ives, 2008, p. 2). Conditions commonly included within this definition include scurvy (resulting from vitamin C deficiency), rickets and osteomalacia (related to vitamin D deficiency), bone loss including osteoporosis, and Paget's disease of bone; clinical examinations of metabolic bone disease may also encompass rarer hereditary metabolic disturbances that are generally less relevant to paleopathologists, except in isolated cases. Clinical data provide the primary source of evidence for metabolic disease processes. However, significant differences in the types of evidence, methodologies, and approaches available to clinicians and to paleopathologists affect the ways in which clinical data can be utilized in paleopathology. Methods of clinical examination that involve directly evaluating or visualizing the skeleton have more obvious application to paleopathology. This includes radiographic imaging methods (Mays, 2008a) and histological techniques, which have grown out of modern standards for the examination of clinical biopsy samples (Turner-Walker and Mays, 2008). Clinical research on bone biology elucidates the underlying mechanisms of disease processes and their skeletal manifestations, and genetic and endocrinological studies have been instrumental in examining controlling and complicating factors in these processes. Clinical case studies provide detailed information about individual disease manifestations and etiological factors, while epidemiological studies outline broader trends at a population level, providing information on disease incidence rates and trends related to factors such as age, sex, and social determinants of health. The availability of detailed patient histories, descriptions of symptoms experienced, soft tissue evidence for disease, and comprehensive biochemical and genetic laboratory testing augments clinicians' ability to recognize and diagnose metabolic conditions; these data may not be directly applicable to paleopathological cases, but they do provide valuable evidence on individuals' lived experiences of disease.

8.2 NEGOTIATING MEDICINE AND ANTHROPOLOGY WITHIN PALEOPATHOLOGY

Paleopathology has matured since the 19th century from a "physician's hobby" to a discipline in its own right (eg, Armelagos, 1997; Grauer, 2008). The balance of influence in paleopathology has shifted throughout the discipline's development, as analyses expanded from focusing almost exclusively on clinical research toward a much broader use of information from multiple sources, including anthropological perspectives (Cook and Powell, 2006). While paleopathologists now tend to be trained as anthropologists rather than as clinicians (Mays, 2012a), contributions from both disciplines remain vital to progress within paleopathology (eg, Buikstra, 2010; Ortner, 2011; Rothschild and Martin, 1993). Clinical knowledge is essential for recognizing evidence of disease processes and for updating diagnostic criteria based on relevant advances in clinical literature, while anthropological knowledge is essential for contextualizing and interpreting disease in past populations (Buikstra et al., 2011; Goodman, 1993; Grauer, 2008).

While efforts to improve consistency and transparency in paleopathological recording continue (eg, Appleby et al., 2015), progress within paleopathology is often conceptualized as a movement away from an exclusive focus on description and diagnosis toward applying paleopathological information to larger-scale problems (Armelagos and Van Gerven, 2003; Grauer, 2008; Mays, 2012a; Wright and Yoder, 2003). The latter approach is associated with meaningful interpretation and with problem-oriented research (Knudson and Stojanowski, 2008; Ortner, 2011). Contextualized bioarchaeological analysis imparts greater meaning to interpretations of metabolic bone disease in the past (Knüsel, 2010), as does the explicit integration of anthropological theory (eg, Agarwal, 2012).

During the initial development of biocultural and bioarchaeological perspectives, clinical approaches were characterized as individual in scale, focused entirely on description and diagnosis, and lacking meaningful interpretation (Meiklejohn and Zvelebil, 1991). Biocultural approaches were contextualized, comprehensive, corresponded more closely with lived experience, and involved problem-oriented research that applied paleopathological data to broader, anthropologically significant questions (Zimmerman and Kelley, 1982). This dichotomy sometimes persists in the anthropological literature (eg, Armelagos and Van Gerven, 2003; Zuckerman and Armelagos, 2011), but ultimately reflects a narrow conception of clinical research that equates the clinical approach with descriptive case studies. This does not acknowledge the enormous growth and burgeoning importance of clinical epidemiological research, in which the gold standard for modern evidence-based medicine involves statistical investigation of disease patterns in large numbers of patients, and overlooks the value that case studies can have for communicating information on uncommon conditions (Mays, 2012a,b). Highlighting connections between perceived analytical problems within paleopathology and its relationship with medicine (Zuckerman and Armelagos, 2011) must be done carefully so as not to promote an inaccurate characterization of clinical approaches, potentially widening the gap between anthropological subfields (Goodman and Leatherman, 1998) and discouraging the development of productive biocultural and bioarchaeological discourse. It is important to recognize that clinical data on the etiology and functional consequences of metabolic conditions affecting the skeleton have been an essential part of many meaningful bioarchaeological interpretations of disease experience and of the implications of disease expression for sociocultural and lifestyle factors in the past (eg, Agarwal et al., 2004; Agarwal and Grynpas, 2009; Mays et al., 2013; Van der Merwe et al., 2010).

8.3 USES OF CLINICAL DATA: PALEOPATHOLOGICAL ANALYSES OF METABOLIC BONE DISEASE

Paleopathological investigations of metabolic bone disease use clinical data to discuss symptoms, skeletal manifestations, and pathophysiology of disease processes, to elucidate etiological factors related to disease occurrence in the present and the past, to discuss functional outcomes, consequences, and disease experiences, and to impart a dimension of time to the static skeletal picture of disease. Time is accessed through clinical evidence for dynamic aspects of disease expression, including severity, manifestations of different disease stages, and differences between active and healed disease (Brickley et al., 2010). Archaeological skeletons present a cumulative picture of disease experience over the life course, as represented at the moment of death (Ortner, 2011). So, as dynamic measures of bone formation and resorption can only be measured in living patients, insights into the dynamic state of osteological processes that can be gained in paleopathology are based on information gleaned from clinical observations of these processes (Cho and Stout, 2003).

Accurate diagnoses, dependent on clinically established associations of skeletal manifestations with other markers of disease, are fundamental to paleopathological analyses of metabolic bone disease (Grauer, 2008; Waldron, 2009). This process of biomedical clinical analogy

(Klepinger, 1983) provides a permanent role for clinical data in paleo-pathology. At the most basic level, diagnosis involves distinguishing abnormal change from normal structure, as defined using modern medical data (Huss-Ashmore et al., 1982). Clinical diagnoses begin with clusters of symptoms that can be connected to known syndromes; given the combination of symptoms described by a patient, physicians determine which syndrome is likely represented, and attempt to confirm this preliminary diagnosis through laboratory and other diagnostic techniques (Coe and Favus, 2002). Understanding how symptoms are connected within a syndrome requires a complete understanding of the underlying disease process (Schultz, 2001). Similarly, paleopatho-logical diagnosis can best be accomplished by recognizing and connect-ing skeletal features of disease through the underlying mechanism, rather than matching individual lesion appearances with reference samples (Aufderheide and Rodríguez-Martín, 1998; Ortner, 2003, p. 48, 2011). Thorough differential diagnoses systematically consider the level of clinical and contextual support for several alternatives, and employ multiple types of evidence to differentiate nonspecific lesions (Schultz, 2001).

Paleopathological analyses are also informed by clinical priorities and results, which may serve as the basis for hypotheses (Mays, 2008b). Expectations for etiological associations, severity, and trends of occur-rence by age and sex in the past may be based on modern patterns and modern medical paradigms (eg, Agarwal et al., 2004; Brickley and Agarwal, 2003; Mays, 2003; Mays et al., 2006; Stirland, 1991), making it important to recognize the ways that this can limit interpretations of metabolic disease in past societies. For example, Agarwal (2012) demonstrates that patterns of bone maintenance in a British medieval skeletal sample are not constrained by senescence and menopause, as predicted by biomedical models. Therefore, in automatically dividing bioarchaeological samples by sex as the first step in analyzing bone loss, other sources of variation may be underestimated or even missed altogether (Agarwal, 2012).

8.4 CLINICAL DATA AND PALEOPATHOLOGY: AREAS OF DISCONNECT

The majority of clinical information is not directly applicable to paleopathology, but must be adapted into criteria appropriate for diagnosing metabolic conditions in dry bone (Waldron, 2009, pp. 4–6). Developing specific dry bone diagnostic criteria isolates indicators that are best suited to the evidence available while retaining an important link with clinical data (see Mays, 2012a). This link is most effectively preserved by retaining and applying clinically accepted terminology and definitions, which minimizes confusion in the transfer of clinical information to paleopathological analyses and enables productive dialogue (Cook and Powell, 2006; Grauer, 2008; Ragsdale and Lehmer, 2012). In adapting entire classificatory systems, differences in the objectives of clinical and paleopathological study must be accounted for (Ortner, 2011). A system developed for treating living patients is unlikely to be entirely appropriate for paleopathological samples of individuals who have long been dead and buried. In some ways, clinical and paleopathological understandings of skeletal involvement in metabolic disease differ, as the clinical picture of a condition includes soft tissue, biochemical, and in vivo radiographic features whereas paleopathology relies on dry bone. Despite this limitation, the primacy of skeletal changes in metabolic bone diseases may make paleopathological and clinical conceptions of this category of disorders more directly comparable to one another than is the case for other types of disease.

Clinical and paleopathological analyses utilize many of the same diagnostic methods, including radiography, histology, and clinical imaging technologies, but their applications and levels of importance may vary depending on the type and utility of other methods available to assess evidence for disease (Mays, 2012a; Ortner, 2011). Histological examination of bone using light or scanning electron microscopy is used to interpret pathological structural changes in the skeleton. Since modern clinicians avoid taking invasive and painful samples unless they are absolutely necessary for diagnosis (Mays, 2012a), clinically diagnosed comparative material is more likely to be restricted to historical samples or to the few skeletal conditions for which these analyses remain routine, including renal osteodystrophy (Mays and Turner-Walker, 2008). Radiography, on the other hand, represents the primary clinical strategy for directly accessing information on the skeleton, and is important for investigating bone diseases. Radiographic criteria can often be more directly applied to paleopathology than gross or microscopic criteria for which relevant clinical evidence differs more significantly (Mays, 2008c).

Clinical diagnoses that use skeletal features do so in combination with many other sources of evidence for disease processes that may have greater diagnostic value than features visible in dry bone. For example, vitamin D deficiency can be easily diagnosed biochemically from a blood sample, enabling early detection of disease and negating the need for more invasive procedures such as skeletal biopsy (Brickley and Ives, 2008). Many clinical diagnoses therefore rely on information that is inaccessible in archaeological skeletal material, decreasing the applicability of modern clinical methods in paleopathological diagnosis and encouraging reliance on older clinical research to bridge the gap between the two. Based on modern clinical data, it is evident that "classic" manifestations of disease processes represent a small fraction of the typical distribution of cases (Miller et al., 1996; Ortner, 2011). There is significant variation in disease expression, not all of which is described clinically, and even less of which is described in the clinical literature in terms of features that can be detected in dry bone.

Many uses of clinical data in paleopathological contexts are impacted by the nature of evidence available to clinicians and to paleopathologists. Preservation and potential diagenetic alterations following burial can affect bone structure and lesion appearance. In metabolic diseases bone quantity and quality are often compromised, making elements more vulnerable to fragmentation (Brickley et al., 2005). The adaptation of clinical diagnostic criteria for use in paleopathology must therefore consider how gross, radiographic, and microscopic lesion appearances may be masked, erased, or mimicked by taphonomic processes (Pfeiffer, 2000). It is also necessary to consider differences in disease experience between archaeological individuals and those described in clinical cases or contained in historical pathology collections, and how these might affect the ability to recognize evidence for disease in the past. Most modern clinical cases are prevented from running a full or natural course, and lesion appearance may be altered by treatment or milder than would be expected if the disease had been allowed to progress (Zimmerman and Kelley, 1982). This is where historical medical literature, documenting the natural course of disease prior to the development of effective treatments, may be particularly useful. Some recent cases of disease, diagnosed late due to lack of clinical experience with conditions that are rare in modern developed countries, such as scurvy and severe rickets (eg, Noordin et al., 2012), may also bear closer resemblance to ancient cases.

8.5 DIAGNOSING METABOLIC DISEASE IN THE PAST

Despite difficulties associated with adapting clinical criteria to diagnoses using dry bone, many clinically documented features of metabolic conditions affecting the skeleton are available for application to paleopathological analyses. As well, clinical studies are invaluable in elucidating details of underlying metabolic disturbances and the processes through which they affect the skeleton. Despite the suggestion of various standardized criteria, such as the operational definitions proposed by Waldron (2009), paleopathological diagnoses vary appreciably in terms of the methods and criteria applied. Significant differences of opinion exist regarding how much and what types of clinical data are required to securely establish links between skeletal lesions and specific diagnoses of metabolic bone disease.

One end of this scale is represented by paleopathological analyses of vitamin D deficiency rickets and osteomalacia. Diagnoses of these conditions in archaeological skeletal material are generally directly linked with clinical descriptions of skeletal manifestations and available radiographic data (Brickley and Ives, 2008; Ortner, 2003). Modern medicine recognizes bone as a primary site of abnormalities when vitamin D and calcium metabolism are disturbed due to the integral role of the skeleton in calcium metabolism and its importance as a primary site of action of vitamin D. Skeletal features of rickets including bowing deformities, expanded metaphyses, flaring at the costochondral rib ends, and features of osteomalacia such as pseudofractures, are visible on clinical radiographs (Brickley and Ives, 2008). Accordingly, direct clinical evidence is available to associate skeletal lesions with vitamin D deficiency in both adults and children. In this case, disease manifestations relevant to paleopathologists and to clinicians align, and both utilize methods like radiography that allow skeletal manifestations to be clearly identified. An abundance of historical (eg, Holt, 1908; Jaffe, 1972, 1975) and modern (eg, Meunier and Chapuy, 2005; Pettifor, 2003; Pitt, 2002; Priemel et al., 2010; Reginato and Coquia, 2003) clinical data on macroscopic, radiographic, and histological manifestations of vitamin D deficiency rickets and osteomalacia exist that directly relate to features identifiable in archaeological material.

Conversely, paleopathological recognition of scurvy in juvenile remains tends to rely on indirect clinical evidence. Modern medical understandings of this condition place primary emphasis on defects in collagen synthesis, making the role of the skeleton less central in scurvy than in vitamin D deficiency. Clinical diagnosis of scurvy relies on soft tissue features (Huss-Ashmore et al., 1982). While skeletal changes are recognized clinically, the disease is known to primarily affect connective tissue, meaning that skeletal manifestations are largely secondary.

Differences in the types of evidence available to paleopathologists and clinicians for diagnosing scurvy are also related to the variation in priorities between those studying human remains and those treating living patients, especially relating to differential applications of radiographic methods. As a result of concerns over exposure to radiation, clinicians only radiograph patients when necessary, and only image the portion of the body in which symptoms are reported. Radiographic evidence for the total clinical pattern of skeletal involvement in the body is typically lacking (Ortner, 1991). Paleopathologists have proposed abnormal porosity in the skull as a criterion for skeletal diagnoses of scurvy. However, this is an area of the body that clinicians avoid exposing to X-ray. Since direct clinical evidence for this feature is lacking, paleopathologists have relied on indirect evidence, theoretically explaining how clinically observed soft tissue lesions, mainly swelling and redness in the temporal region, might affect the skeleton in the form of porosity in various areas of the skull, particularly the greater wing of the sphenoid (Ortner and Ericksen, 1997). The physiological reasoning used to support this association, worked through in minute detail by Ortner and Ericksen (1997), elucidates a rather convincing mechanism behind the formation of skeletal changes. The inferred connection between soft tissue lesions associated with chronic bleeding, inflammation, and consequent bone porosity is supported indirectly by established clinical connections between these processes. However, others have emphasized that in order for these criteria to be used in rigorous diagnoses, the proposed link must be confirmed by direct and reliable clinical evidence (Melikian and Waldron, 2003; Waldron, 2009), or at the very least cranial lesions must be shown to co-occur with more securely established manifestations such as clinical radiological indicators, periosteal new bone, and abnormal porosity in the long bones (Stark, 2014). While one documented historical medical case does exist and shows cranial porosity (Ortner, 2011), this individual was originally diagnosed as having congenital syphilis, and the diagnosis was retrospectively changed to scurvy. Cranial porosity can be productively viewed as a potential manifestation of scurvy in the juvenile skeleton, but until more direct clinical evidence is available to support this linkage, it seems prudent to avoid utilizing this feature as a major determinant for diagnoses.

Subsequent researchers have variously incorporated criteria suggested by Ortner and Ericksen (1997). Despite the relatively conservative attitude originally displayed toward diagnosing scurvy based on porosity (Ortner and Ericksen, 1997), subsequent papers (Ortner et al., 1999, 2001; Trainer, 2012) have presented porosity on the greater wing of the sphenoid as pathognomonic of scurvy, and some have gone so far as to eliminate skeletal individuals from an analysis if they are missing this element. Some paleopathological diagnoses of scurvy in the skeleton are therefore reliant on a single criterion based upon indirect clinical supporting evidence, allowing assumptions of its validity to dictate not only interpretations but also methodology and research design. Ortner et al.'s (1999) use of the term "pathognomonic" implies a very high level of certainty in their diagnoses of scurvy, despite the use of qualifying terminology like "probable" and "most likely" in other areas of the paper. Other analyses acknowledge the dangers of overreliance on this single skeletal indicator, considering it in combination with several other skeletal features and maintaining a level of caution in diagnosis (eg, Brickley and Ives, 2006; Brown and Ortner, 2011; Geber and Murphy, 2012; Lewis, 2010; Mays, 2008c), often incorporating thorough differential diagnoses that consider other etiological possibilities. Melikian and Waldron (2003) go so far as to conclude that certain diagnosis based on cranial porosity is not possible. Ortner (2003, pp. 390−393) suggests that further research will be able to confirm the linkage suggested from indirect evidence but maintains that a diagnosis can be made on the basis of such evidence if carefully considered; on the other hand, Waldron (2009) rejects these criteria outright until direct evidence is provided. Opinion regarding the security of paleopathological diagnoses of scurvy based indirectly on clinical data therefore varies from confident (Ortner et al., 1999, 2001) to cautious (Waldron, 2009). While well-reasoned manifestations of scurvy like abnormal cranial porosity should be considered in the overall skeletal picture of disease, they should not be relied upon to support the weight of diagnoses, and certainly not to determine methodology.

In concordance with the use of both direct and indirect clinical evidence to evaluate skeletal manifestations, the paleopathological literature reveals clear trends in how diagnostic features supported by clinical information are referenced, either by directly citing clinical studies or by indirectly using clinical data collated by paleopathological reference texts or analyses. Following the initial paleopathological association of clinical manifestations of scurvy indirectly to dry bone manifestations (Ortner and Ericksen, 1997), some analyses cite this and subsequent paleopathological papers (eg, Ortner et al., 1999, 2001) rather than directly engaging with clinical literature (eg, Bourbou, 2003; Buckley, 2000; Lambert, 2006; Lewis, 2002, 2010; Ortner et al., 2007; Salis et al., 2005; Stirland, 2000). This is understandable, particularly given the lack of direct clinical corroboration for this feature; however, if clinical data have not been rigorously applied in the cited studies then the certainty of subsequent diagnoses may be affected.

On the other hand, many paleopathological studies, especially those dealing with diagnostic criteria that are closely linked to clinical evidence, directly cite modern medical studies of metabolic bone disease (eg, Brickley and Agarwal, 2003; Brickley and Ives, 2008; Mays, 2003, 2010; Pinto and Stout, 2010). Clinical data tend to be cited directly when describing new or unusual manifestations that have not been previously documented in paleopathological cases of disease, such as putative scorbutic lesions associated with involvement of the scapula (Brickley and Ives, 2006) or ilium (Brown and Ortner, 2011), proliferation of new bone around the foramina rotundi (Geber and Murphy, 2012), or subdural hemorrhage (Mays, 2008c). This trend is also reflected in the literature on vitamin D deficiency, where clinical data are often directly referenced when documenting disease manifestations rarely observed paleopathologically (eg, Blondiaux et al., 2002; Formicola, 1995; Mays et al., 2006; Mays and Turner-Walker, 2008; Pfeiffer and Crowder, 2004), including lesions in adults (Brickley et al., 2007).

8.6 INTEGRATING CLINICAL AND ANTHROPOLOGICAL PERSPECTIVES

Clinical data also have significant and largely unrecognized potential for application within relevant anthropological theoretical models, including studies of identity and the life course perspective. The biocultural approach, already well established within bioarchaeology, emphasizes the interrelation of biology and culture and the importance of communication in bridging the divide between sciences and humanities (Knüsel, 2010). Explicit engagement in identity studies has developed within bioarchaeology along with increasing recognition that meaningful interpretation can take place at both individual and population levels (eg, Armelagos, 2003; Knudson and Stojanowski, 2008). Given the necessary role of individuals within populations (Buikstra et al., 2011), examining the two levels in concert with one another may be particularly valuable. The cultural relevance of biological processes, including disease, relates to how socially meaningful identity groups differentially experience these conditions, and how these experiences become embodied in the skeleton (Fausto-Sterling, 2005). Clinical descriptions of patients' lived experiences identify the embodied effects of disease processes, as well as how these physical—including skeletal—manifestations relate to symptoms described by an individual during the course of disease and to the severity of the disease process itself. For example, a study by Palkovich (2012) examines the case of a 14th-century Puebloan woman with evidence for severe impairment from childhood rickets, including severe bending deformities and poor muscle development in both upper and lower limbs. Palkovich (2012) discusses ways in which residual rickets may have limited this individual's everyday life as an adult, including limitations to her ability to participate in physically demanding chores typical of the ancestral Puebloan lifestyle, but also how her completely typical burial treatment provides no evidence for differential treatment despite obvious physical impairment. In this case, clinical information regarding potential lasting functional consequences of rickets can be combined with archaeological evidence for potential social roles to explore aspects of individual identity in the past (Palkovich, 2012).

Clinical information on disease progression in relation to processes of growth, aging, and reproductive function can also contribute to paleopathological understandings of metabolic bone disease using a life course approach. This theoretical model conceptualizes the body as a material object produced over the course of an individual's life through biologically meaningful and socially defined actions (Sofaer, 2006a,b). Integrating clinical data could be especially significant in connecting rickets with growth processes, osteomalacia and bone maintenance with pregnancy and lactation, and bone loss with aging. For example, several studies of osteoporosis in archaeological material from Britain incorporate clinical evidence for the effects of pregnancy, lactation, or age-related changes on the skeleton, and focus on how the cumulative product of gendered life-history experiences constructs the skeleton and explains changes in bone status observed in individuals at different stages of the life course (Agarwal, 2012; Mays, 1996, 2000, 2001, 2006).

Paleopathological evidence for metabolic bone disease has been used extensively to provide meaningful information on life in the past. Clinical data, technologies, and approaches have contributed significantly to paleopathological understandings of metabolic bone disease in terms of recognition, diagnosis, and interpretation, and have the potential to contribute to theoretical understandings as well. However, the tendency to reference paleopathological rather than clinical studies for diagnostic criteria that are more "established" paleopathologically reduces direct engagement with clinical information, and may endanger these essential understandings of pathological processes and their relationship with skeletal lesions. There are significant areas of disconnect between clinical and paleopathological evidence and approaches; this is true not only for metabolic bone disease, but also for other conditions relevant to paleopathologists including infectious disease. Despite these differences, research designs in medical and paleopathological research are fundamentally similar. The gold standard for modern evidence-based medicine involves statistical examination of disease patterns in large numbers of patients (Mays, 2012a,b), similar to the population-level studies prioritized by bioarchaeologists. Excellent paleopathological research will continue to apply clinical data as directly as possible, while incorporating anthropological perspectives to contextualize and deepen interpretations.

Bioarchaeological examinations of skeletal evidence for metabolic bone diseases provide important insight into the occurrence of metabolic conditions in environments that both resemble and differ from modern contexts. As paleopathologists continue to negotiate the boundaries between dichotomized elements, maintaining close correspondence with the research goals and methods of clinicians will facilitate mutual engagement with the potential to expand understandings of metabolic disease processes both in the present and in the past.

Paleopathology is in a unique position to bridge the divide between science and art by integrating clinical data with anthropological theoretical perspectives to answer questions with broad contemporary relevance both to medicine and to anthropology.

REFERENCES

Agarwal, S.C., 2012. The past of sex, gender, and health: bioarchaeology of the aging skeleton. Am. Anthropol. 114, 322–335.

Agarwal, S.C., Grynpas, M.D., 2009. Measuring and interpreting age-related loss of vertebral bone mineral density in a medieval population. Am. J. Phys. Anthropol. 139, 244–252.

Agarwal, S.C., Dumitriu, M., Tomlinson, G.A., Grynpas, M.D., 2004. Medieval trabecular bone architecture: the influence of age, sex, and lifestyle. Am. J. Phys. Anthropol. 124, 33–44.

Appleby, J., Thomas, R., Buikstra, J., 2015. Increasing confidence in paleopathological diagnosis—application of the Istanbul terminological framework. Int. J. Palaeopath. 8, 19–21.

Armelagos, G.J., 1997. Paleopathology. In: Frank, S. (Ed.), History of Physical Anthropology: An Encyclopedia. Garland Publishing, New York, NY, pp. 790–796.

Armelagos, G.J., 2003. Bioarchaeology as anthropology. Arch. Papers Anthropol. Assoc. 13, 27–40.

Armelagos, G.J., Van Gerven, D.P., 2003. A century of skeletal biology and paleopathology: contrasts, contradictions, and conflicts. Am. Anthropol. 105, 53–64.

Aufderheide, A.C., Rodríguez-Martín, C., 1998. The Cambridge Encyclopedia of Human Paleopathology. Cambridge University Press, Cambridge, MA.

Blondiaux, G., Blondiaux, J., Secousse, F., Cotton, A., Danze, P.-M., Flipo, R.-M., 2002. Rickets and child abuse: the case of a two year old girl from the 4th century in Lisieux (Normandy). Int. J. Osteoarchaol. 12, 209–215.

Bourbou, C., 2003. Health patterns of proto-Byzantine populations (6th-7th centuries AD) in south Greece: the cases of Eleutherna (Crete) and Messene (Peloponnese). Int. J. Osteoarchaol. 13, 303–313.

Brickley, M., Agarwal, S.C., 2003. Techniques for the investigation of age-related bone loss and osteoporosis in archaeological bone. In: Agarwal, S.C., Stout, S.D. (Eds.), Bone Loss and Osteoporosis: An Anthropological Perspective. Kluwer Academic/Plenum Publishers, New York, NY, pp. 157–172.

Brickley, M., Ives, R., 2006. Skeletal manifestations of infantile scurvy. Am. J. Phys. Anthropol. 129, 163–172.

Brickley, M., Ives, R., 2008. The Bioarchaeology of Metabolic Bone Disease. Academic Press, Oxford.

Brickley, M., Mays, S., Ives, R., 2005. Skeletal manifestations of vitamin D deficiency osteomalacia in documented historical collections. Int. J. Osteoarchaol. 15, 389–403.

Brickley, M., Mays, S., Ives, R., 2007. An investigation of skeletal indicators of vitamin D deficiency in adults: effective markers for interpreting past living conditions and pollution levels in 18th and 19th century Birmingham, England. Am. J. Phys. Anthropol. 132, 67–79.

Brickley, M., Mays, S., Ives, R., 2010. Evaluation and interpretation of residual rickets deformities in adults. Int. J. Osteoarchaol. 20, 54–66.

Brown, M., Ortner, D.J., 2011. Childhood scurvy in a medieval burial from Macvanska Mitrovica, Serbia. Int. J. Osteoarchaeol. 21, 197–207.

Buckley, H.R., 2000. Subadult health and disease in prehistoric Tonga, Polynesia. Am. J. Phys. Anthropol. 113, 481–505.

Buikstra, J.E., 2010. Paleopathology: a contemporary perspective. In: Larsen, C.S. (Ed.), A Companion to Biological Anthropology. Wiley Blackwell, Malden, pp. 395–411.

Buikstra, J.E., Baadsgaard, A., Boutin, A.T., 2011. Introduction. In: Baadsgaard, A., Boutin, A. T., Buikstra, J.E. (Eds.), Breathing New Life into the Evidence of Death: Contemporary Approaches to Bioarchaeology. School for Advanced Research Press, Santa Fe, pp. 3–26.

Bush, H., Zvelebil, M., 1991. Pathology and health in past societies: an introduction. In: Bush, H., Zvelebil, M. (Eds.), Health in Past Societies: Biocultural Interpretations of Human Skeletal Remains in Archaeological Contexts. Tempvs Reparatvm, Oxford, pp. 3–10.

Cho, H., Stout, S.D., 2003. Bone remodeling and age-associated bone loss in the past: a histomorphometric analysis of the Imperial Roman skeletal population of Isola Sacra. In: Agarwal, S.C., Stout, S.D. (Eds.), Bone Loss and Osteoporosis: An Anthropological Perspective. Kluwer Academic/Plenum Publishers, New York, NY, pp. 207–228.

Coe, F.L., Favus, M.J., 2002. Clinical and laboratory approach to the patient with disorders of bone and mineral metabolism. In: Coe, F.L., Favus, M.J. (Eds.), Disorders of Bone and Mineral Metabolism, second ed. Lippincott Williams & Wilkins, Philadelphia, PA, pp. 399–405.

Cook, D.C., Powell, M.L., 2006. The evolution of American paleopathology. In: Buikstra, J.E., Beck, L.A. (Eds.), Bioarchaeology: The Contextual Analysis of Human Remains. Elsevier, Burlington, CA, pp. 281–322.

Fausto-Sterling, A., 2005. The bare bones of sex: Part 1—sex and gender. Signs 30, 1491–1527.

Formicola, V., 1995. X-linked hypophosphatemic rickets: a probable Upper Paleolithic case. Am. J. Phys. Anthropol. 98, 403–409.

Geber, J., Murphy, E., 2012. Scurvy in the great Irish famine: evidence of vitamin C deficiency from a mid-19th century skeletal population. Am. J. Phys. Anthropol. 148, 512–524.

Goodman, A.H., 1993. On the interpretation of health from skeletal remains. Curr. Anthropol. 34, 281–288.

Goodman, A.H., Leatherman, T.L., 1998. Traversing the chasm between biology and culture: an introduction. In: Goodman, A.H., Leatherman, T.L. (Eds.), Building a New Biocultural Synthesis: Political-Economic Perspectives on Human Biology. The University of Michigan Press, Ann Arbor, MI, pp. 3–42.

Grauer, A.L., 2008. Macroscopic analysis and data collection in paleopathology. In: Pinhasi, R., Mays, S. (Eds.), Advances in Human Palaeopathology. John Wiley & Sons, Chichester, pp. 57–76.

Holt, L.E., 1908. The Diseases of Infancy and Childhood, fourth ed. D Appleton and Company, New York, NY.

Huss-Ashmore, R., Goodman, A.H., Armelagos, G.J., 1982. Nutritional inference from paleopathology. Adv. Archaeol. Meth. Theory 5, 395–474.

Jaffe, H.L., 1972. Metabolic Degenerative, and Inflammatory Diseases of Bones and Joints. Lea & Febiger, Philadelphia, PA.

Jaffe, H.L., 1975. Rickets and osteomalacia. In: Jaffe, H.L. (Ed.), Metabolic, Degenerative, and Inflammatory Diseases of Bones and Joints. Lea & Febiger, Philadephia, PA, pp. 381–447.

Klepinger, L.L., 1983. Differential diagnosis in paleopathology and the concept of disease evolution. Med. Anthropol. 7, 73–77.

Knudson, K.J., Stojanowski, C.M., 2008. New directions in bioarchaeology: recent contributions to the study of human social identities. J. Archaeol. Res 16, 397–432.

Knüsel, C.J., 2010. Bioarchaeology: a synthetic approach. Bull. Mém. Soc. Anthropol. Paris 22, 62–73.

Lambert, P.M., 2006. Infectious disease among enslaved African Americans at Eaton's Estate, Warren County, North Carolina, ca. 1830-1850. Mem. Inst. Oswaldo Cruz 101 (SII), 107–117.

Lewis, M., 2002. Impact of industrialization: comparative study of child health in four sites from medieval and postmedieval England (A.D. 850-1859). Am. J. Phys. Anthropol. 119, 211–223.

Lewis, M., 2010. Life and death in a civitas capital: metabolic disease and trauma in the children from late Roman Dorchester, Dorset. Am. J. Phys. Anthropol. 142, 405–416.

Mays, S., 1996. Age-dependent cortical bone loss in a medieval population. Int. J. Osteoarchaeol. 6, 144–154.

Mays, S., 2000. Age-dependent cortical bone loss in women from 19th and early 19th century London. Am. J. Phys. Anthropol. 112, 349–361.

Mays, S., 2001. Effects of age and occupation on cortical bone in a group of 18th-19th century British men. Am. J. Phys. Anthropol. 116, 34–44.

Mays, S., 2003. The rise and fall of rickets in England. In: Murphy, P., Wiltshire, P.E.J. (Eds.), The Environmental Archaeology of Industry. Oxbow Books, Oxford, pp. 144–153.

Mays, S., 2006. Age-related cortical bone loss in women from a 3rd-4th century AD population from England. Am. J. Phys. Anthropol. 129, 518–528.

Mays, S., 2008a. Radiography and allied techniques in the paleopathology of skeletal remains. In: Pinhasi, R., Mays, S. (Eds.), Advances in Human Palaeopathology. John Wiley & Sons, Chichester, pp. 77–100.

Mays, S., 2008b. Metabolic bone disease. In: Pinhasi, R., Mays, S. (Eds.), Advances in Human Paleopathology. John Wiley & Sons, Chichester, pp. 215–252.

Mays, S., 2008c. A likely case of scurvy from early Bronze Age Britain. Int. J. Osteoarchaeol. 18, 178–187.

Mays, S., 2010. Archaeological skeletons support a northwest European origin for Paget's disease of bone. J. Bone Miner. Res. 25, 1839–1841.

Mays, S., 2012a. The relationship between paleopathology and the clinical sciences. In: Grauer, A.L. (Ed.), A Companion to Paleopathology. Wiley-Blackwell, Oxford, pp. 285–309.

Mays, S., 2012b. The impact of case reports relative to other types of publication in palaeopathology. Int. J. Osteoarchaeol. 22, 81–85.

Mays, S., Turner-Walker, G., 2008. A possible case of renal osteodystrophy in a skeleton from medieval Wharram Percy, England. Int. J. Osteoarchaeol. 18, 307–316.

Mays, S., Brickley, M., Ives, R., 2006. Skeletal manifestations of rickets in infants and young children in a historic population from England. Am. J. Phys. Anthropol. 129, 362–374.

Mays, S., Maat, G.J.R., De Boer, H.H., 2013. Scurvy as a factor in the loss of the 1845 Franklin expedition to the Arctic: a reconsideration. Int. J. Osteoarchaeol. 25, 334–344.

Meiklejohn, C., Zvelebil, M., 1991. Health status of European populations at the agricultural transition and the implications for the adoption of farming. In: Bush, H., Zvelebil, M. (Eds.), Health in Past Societies: Biocultural Interpretations of Human Skeletal Remains in Archaeological Contexts. Tempvs Reparatvm, Oxford, pp. 129–145.

Melikian, M., Waldron, R., 2003. An examination of skulls from two British sites for possible evidence of scurvy. Int. J. Osteoarchaeol. 13, 207–212.

Meunier, P.J., Chapuy, M.C., 2005. Vitamin D insufficiency in adults and the elderly. In: Feldman, D., Pike, J.W., Glorieux, F.H. (Eds.), Vitamin D, second ed. Elsevier Academic Press, San Diego, CA, pp. 1085–1100.

Miller, E., Ragsdale, B.D., Ortner, D.J., 1996. Accuracy in dry bone diagnosis: a comment on palaeopathological methods. Int. J. Osteoarchaeol. 6, 221–229.

Noordin, S., Baloch, N., Salat, M.S., Memon, A.R., Ahman, T., 2012. Skeletal manifestations of scurvy: a case report from Dubai. Case Rep. Orthop. 2012. Available from: http://dx.doi.org/10.1155/2012/624628.

Ortner, D.J., 1991. Theoretical and methodological issues in paleopathology. In: Ortner, D.J., Aufderheide, A.C. (Eds.), Human Paleopathology: Current Syntheses and Future Options. Smithsonian Institution Press, Washington, DC, pp. 5–11.

Ortner, D.J., 2003. Identification of Pathological Conditions in Human Skeletal Remains. Academic Press, San Diego, CA.

Ortner, D.J., 2011. Human skeletal paleopathology. Int. J. Paleopathol. 1, 4–11.

Ortner, D.J., Ericksen, M.F., 1997. Bone changes in the human skull probably resulting from scurvy in infancy and childhood. Int. J. Osteoarchaeol. 7, 212–220.

Ortner, D.J., Kimmerle, E.H., Diez, M., 1999. Probable evidence of scurvy in subadults from archeological sites in Peru. Am. J. Phys. Anthropol. 108, 321–331.

Ortner, D.J., Butler, W., Cafarella, J., Milligan, L., 2001. Evidence of probable scurvy in subadults from archeological sites in North America. Am. J. Phys. Anthropol. 1114, 343–351.

Ortner, D.J., Garofalo, E.M., Zuckerman, M.K., 2007. The EB IA burials of Bâb edh-Dhrâ', Jordan: bioarchaeological evidence of metabolic disease. In: Faerman, M., Horwitz, L.K., Kahana, T., Zilberman, U. (Eds.), Faces from the Past: Diachronic Patterns in the Biology of Human Populations from the Eastern Mediterranean. Papers in Honour of Patricia Smith. Archeopress, Oxford, pp. 181–194.

Palkovich, A.M., 2012. Reading a life: a fourteenth-century ancestral Puebloan woman. In: Stodder, A.L., Palkovich, A.M. (Eds.), The Bioarchaeology of Individuals. University Press of Florida, Gainsville, pp. 242–254.

Pettifor, J.M., 2003. Nutritional rickets. In: Glorieux, F.H., Pettifor, J.M., Jüppner, H. (Eds.), Pediatric Bone: Biology and Diseases. Academic Press, San Diego, CA, pp. 541–566.

Pfeiffer, S., 2000. Palaeohistology: health and disease. In: Katzenberg, M.A., Saunders, S.R. (Eds.), Biological Anthropology of the Human Skeleton. Wiley-Liss, New York, NY, pp. 287–302.

Pfeiffer, S., Crowder, C., 2004. An ill child among Mid-Holocene foragers of southern Africa. Am. J. Phys. Anthropol. 123, 23–29.

Pinto, D.C., Stout, S.D., 2010. Paget's disease in pre-contact Florida? Revisiting the Briarwoods site in gulf coast Florida. Int. J. Osteoarchaeol. 20, 572–578.

Pitt, M.J., 2002. Rickets and osteomalacia. In: Resnick, D. (Ed.), Diagnosis of Bone and Joint Disorders, fourth ed. WB Saunders, Philadelphia, PA, pp. 1901–1945.

Priemel, M., von Domarus, C., Klatte, T.O., Kessler, S., Schlie, J., Meier, S., et al., 2010. Bone mineralization defects and vitamin D deficiency: histomorphometric analysis of iliac crest bone biopsies and circulating 25-hydroxyvitamin D in 675 patients. J. Bone Miner. Res. 25, 305–312.

Ragsdale, B.D., Lehmer, L.M., 2012. A knowledge of bone at the cellular (histological) level is essential to paleopathology. In: Grauer, A.L. (Ed.), A Companion to Paleopathology. Wiley-Blackwell, Oxford, pp. 225–249.

Reginato, A.J., Coquia, J.A., 2003. Musculoskeletal manifestations of osteomalacia and rickets. Best Pract. Res. Clin. Rheumatol 17, 1063–1080.

Rothschild, B.M., Martin, L.D., 1993. Paleopathology: Disease in the Fossil Record. CRC Press, Boca Raton.

Salis, N., Dettoni, E.M., Fulcheri, E., Massa, E.R., 2005. Pathological lesions attributable to vitamin deficiency in skeletal remains from Puy St. Pierre (Briancon, France). Int. J. Anthropol. 20, 325–330.

Schultz, M., 2001. Paleohistopathology of bone: a new approach to the study of ancient diseases. Yearbk. Phys. Anthropol. 44, 106–147.

Sofaer, J.R., 2006a. The Body as Material Culture: A Theoretical Osteoarchaeology. Cambridge University Press, Cambridge.

Sofaer, J.R., 2006b. Gender, bioarchaeology and human ontogeny. In: Gowland, R., Knüsel, C. (Eds.), Social Archaeology of Funerary Remains. Oxbow Books, Oxford, pp. 155–167.

Stark, R.J., 2014. A proposed framework for the study of paleopathological cases of subadult scurvy. Int. J. Paleopathol 5, 18–26.

Stirland, A., 1991. Paget's disease (osteitis deformans): a classic case? Int. J. Osteoarchaeol. 1, 173–177.

Stirland, A.J., 2000. Raising the Dead: The Skeleton Crew of King Henry VIII's Great Ship, the Mary Rose. John Wiley & Sons, Chichester.

Trainer, A.K., 2012. Evidence of juvenile scurvy: a case study from the lower Illinois River valley. Further. Perspect. Anthropol. Views World 5, 42–58.

Turner-Walker, G., Mays, S., 2008. Histological studies on ancient bone. In: Pinhasi, R., Mays, S. (Eds.), Advances in Human Palaeopathology. John Wiley & Sons, Chichester, pp. 121–146.

Van der Merwe, A.E., Steyn, M., Maat, G.J.R., 2010. Adult scurvy in skeletal remains of late 19th century mineworkers in Kimberley, South Africa. Int. J. Osteoarchaeol. 20, 307–316.

Waldron, T., 2009. Palaeopathology. Cambridge University Press, New York, NY.

Washburn, S.L., 1951. The new physical anthropology. Trans. N. Y. Acad. Sci. Series II 13, 298–304.

Wright, L.E., Yoder, C.J., 2003. Recent progress in bioarchaeology: approaches to the osteological paradox. J. Archaeol. Res 11, 43–70.

Zimmerman, M.R., Kelley, M.A., 1982. Atlas of Human Paleopathology. Praeger Publishers, New York, NY.

Zuckerman, M.K., Armelagos, G.J., 2011. The origins of biocultural dimensions in bioarchaeology. In: Agarwal, S.C., Glencross, B.A. (Eds.), Social Bioarchaeology. Wiley-Blackwell, Malden, pp. 15–43.

CHAPTER *9*

Uniting Perception and Reality in Human Nutrition: Integration of Qualitative and Quantitative Data to Understand Consumption

A. Holland
Department of Anthropology, McMaster University, Hamilton, ON, Canada

9.1 INTRODUCTION

Nutrition and food consumption practices are gaining increasing attention in the academic community from both health and social sciences, as food has become a locus of health-related discussion in the general population. While food studies are certainly not a new topic, the breadth of new food studies has moved beyond either quantitative nutrition measurement or qualitative, culturally-based food use. Food research has historically treated eating and nutrition as separate spheres that were essentially either social or scientific processes (Johnston, 1987; Macbeth and MacClancy, 2004; Pelto et al., 2000). The emergence of research that adapts a more biosocial approach indicates a recognition that food and eating are complex intertwined processes that are heavily influenced by the social framework in which eating is entrenched (MacClancy and Macbeth, 2004). The meanings associated with a specific food item cannot be separated from the nutritional content of that food because the decision to consume a food can be based—at least partially—on nutrition, but also has consequences for the nutritional adequacy of an individual. As a result, nutrition studies cannot be conducted in the absence of the qualitative context of food, and phenomenological studies of food meanings cannot be divorced from the nutritional outcomes of consumption choices (McGarvey, 2009). Qualitative and quantitative methods, however, generate disparate data types that are designed to measure fundamentally different things. This paper will discuss how qualitative research methods, such as interviews and pile sorts, can be united with a quantitative survey approach to produce a unique answer to a research

Beyond the Bones. DOI: http://dx.doi.org/10.1016/B978-0-12-804601-2.00009-0

question. A case study on perceptions of calcium and vitamin D intake in young adults is used to explore the benefits and challenges of this approach. This paper is not designed to be a thorough review of the case study results and methodology, but instead will provide a reflection on the process of integrating data sets and the methodological and theoretical issues that arise.

9.2 STUDYING FOOD AND NUTRITION

Human nutrition studies are important for assessing the nutritional status of populations, which is necessary for monitoring and maintaining population health. The goal of applied nutrition studies involves identifying adequate patterns of consumption for a variety of nutrients so that interventions can be designed to modify intakes (Becker and Welten, 2001; Briefel et al., 1997; Cook et al., 2000; Creed-Kanashiro et al., 2003). Most research into human nutrition focuses on the evaluation of nutrient intake in comparison to set national dietary reference intakes (DRI) (Atkinson, 2011; McPherson et al., 2000; Rizek and Pao, 1990; Ulijaszek, 2004; Whiting et al., 2011). DRIs are generated by the Institute of Medicine (IOM) and serve to identify thresholds of consumption for individual nutrients based on identified population needs (Atkinson, 2011; Health Canada, 2012). The two most commonly used measures are the recommended dietary allowance (RDA) and the estimated average requirement (EAR), which are the amounts of a nutrient needed to satisfy the requirements for 95% and 50% of a population, respectively (IOM, 2010). While the assessments designed to use these standards provide information on the nutrient gaps of individuals and populations, they do not incorporate the role that individual perceptions play in decisions about nutrition.

Decision-making in regards to nutrition relies not only on food and nutrition knowledge, but also upon individuals' perceptions of their intake and their beliefs about food. Perceptions provide a necessary framework within which nutrition knowledge is understood and food decisions are made (Wilson, 2002). The context of food decision-making serves to explain the observed patterns (MacClancy and Macbeth, 2004). Therefore, in order to holistically interpret the food data that are collected through nutrition studies, it is necessary to understand how and why people make specific food choices (Wilson, 2002). Since one goal of human nutrition studies is to design public education or intervention programs that correct over- or under-consumption (Becker and Welten, 2001; Briefel et al., 1997; Garriguet, 2008), the context in which decisions are made becomes essential for designing effective programs.

9.3 USING A MIXED METHODS APPROACH

Mixed methods research holds a contentious place in anthropological research methodology. While proponents of mixed methods research support it as a third paradigm that draws on the best traits of qualitative and quantitative research, purists feel that the fundamentally different nature of the two types of data make them difficult to integrate (Burke Johnson and Onwuegbuzie, 2004). The nature of the debate centers on the epistemological differences in the roles of objectivity and generalizability between qualitative and quantitative methods (Burke Johnson and Onwuegbuzie, 2004; Johnson et al., 2007; Teddlie and Tashakkori, 2003). The social sciences view behavior and belief as concepts that are in flux, and so they are naturally and necessarily subjective, whereas food and nutrition science is required to conceptualize the phenomena they study as having static and objective components because they are searching for measurable truths (Creswell, 2008). Essentially, qualitative approaches are interested in and often centered around context, whereas most quantitative methods are not (Burke Johnson and Onwuegbuzie, 2004). The positivist stance that drives quantitative research is placed in opposition to the relativism of most qualitative methods.

It is these differences in the underlying goals of the methods that lead to problems in their evaluation and integration. Quantitative standards of validity and reliability are held as the ultimate tests for all research methods and are applied to both qualitative and quantitative studies (de Garine, 2004). Reliability and validity assume that there is an objective truth that can be identified, which is viewed as fundamentally in conflict with the relativism of qualitative methods (Golafshani, 2003). The purpose of a mixed methods approach, therefore, is to encourage a pragmatic blending of the social and mental reality of qualitative methods with the physical tangible reality of quantitative methods (Burke Johnson and Onwuegbuzie, 2004). Using a combination of inductive and deductive reasoning expands the breadth of data that can be gathered and proposes a more holistic way of approaching and answering research questions that is more akin to how individuals and researchers actually behave (Driscoll et al., 2007). This means that mixed methods research has the potential to unite multiple lines of evidence to produce more detailed answers to research questions that reflect the complexity that underlies human life and behavior.

An anthropological mixed methods approach to human nutrition studies offers the ability to combine nutrient data with social context. Hubert (2004) presents the study of nutrition as a nested process using multiple methodologies, where qualitative interviews are used to elicit the social context of food and foodways, and quantitative surveys return information on nutrient intake. Since ideas surrounding food are highly contextualized, Hubert (2004) argues that social data on food is necessary for the interpretation of quantitative variables. This means that effective nutrition studies need to include both traditional nutrient intake measurements and beliefs or perceptions about intake (de Garine, 2004; Hubert, 2004). Measuring nutrient intake is generally a quantitative process done using food frequency questionnaires (FFQ), 24-hour food recalls, or food diaries that use recollection or active measurement of intake to provide quantities of foods that are broken down into specific nutrient constituents (Hubert, 2004; Quandt, 1986; Ulijaszek, 2004). These studies produce an intake value for a specific nutrient that can then be compared to the DRI for that population. Perceptions about food use rely on qualitative approaches that are descriptive in nature and explore the meanings behind food decisions and food choice, such as focus groups, interviews, or pile sorts (Edstrom and Devine, 2001; Quintiliani et al., 2008; Vallianatos and Raine, 2008). Uniting these two methodologies creates the potential to either provide social context for observed quantitative trends in food or nutrient intake, or to use qualitative themes to design effective quantitative tools for large populations.

9.4 THE CASE STUDY: MATERIALS AND METHODS

The case study discussed here used an integrated mixed methods approach concerning the importance that calcium and vitamin D played in food decision-making for Canadian young adults, but was specifically geared to assessing the differences in the actual intake of calcium and vitamin D compared to the perceived intake by young adults. Ethics approval was granted by the McMaster University and Mohawk College Internal Review Boards and written consent was obtained from all participants before participation in the study. Sixty male and female (30 of each gender) young adults (17–30 years old) were first given an FFQ specific to calcium and vitamin D, and then participated in a pile sort activity and an in-depth interview. Participants were recruited on campus and from the community and were required to be within the age range and able to give consent to be in the study. No participants were eliminated and none refused to participate. The young adults represented four different education levels: college (2-year program), university (4-year program), postsecondary graduates, and students who had never attended any postsecondary education. The FFQ was designed and validated on a multiethnic Canadian sample and contained 37 food items related to calcium or vitamin D for which participants were asked to indicate the amount consumed and frequency (Wu et al., 2009). The pile sort activity required participants to sort 32 cards that depicted food items into categories for high, medium, or no calcium and yes or no for vitamin D. The pile sort was developed by the researcher for this study and was field tested on a sample of 15 participants before use in the study. Participants were then asked to explain the rationale for each card choice, which led into an in-depth interview on beliefs about nutrition and food choice. All interviews were conducted by the researcher and included questions such as, "do you get enough calcium/vitamin D?" and "how important is nutrition to your daily life?" The goal of the interviews and pile sorts was to explore the degree of conscious choice young adults exercised in food and micronutrient consumption and to assess their nutrition knowledge as a framework for their informed decision-making. The interview lasted between 45–60 minutes and was audio recorded and later transcribed verbatim. The questions ranged from general discussion about nutrition and health to specific questions about vitamin D and calcium.

Analysis of the FFQ involved calculating an average daily intake for calcium and vitamin D using the equation provided by the IOM for the measurement of individual nutrient intake (IOM, 2000). The resulting value was compared to the EAR, a threshold established for these nutrients as set by the IOM to produce a measure of the individuals that were consuming inadequate amounts of calcium and vitamin D (IOM, 2000). Binary logistic regression and Mann-Whitney U tests were used where appropriate to explore the relationship between age, gender, education, and income on consumption patterns. In order to avoid overestimating the individual requirement for a specific nutrient, the IOM recommends using the EAR (IOM, 2000). Analysis of the interviews and pile sorts followed the method for qualitative content analysis described by Bernard (2011). Thematic analysis was conducted on the transcribed interviews and pile sorts, which used a combination of a priori and new codes that reflected the meanings and beliefs raised by the participants. A priori codes were generated before analysis began by establishing broad codes that related to the research question. For example: "importance of nutrition," "knowledge of calcium and vitamin D," and "health as a priority" were a priori codes designed to help guide interpretation in relation to the specific research question. As analysis progressed, new codes were added as themes emerged through a close reading of the data, such as fitness, body image, and individual responsibility. Once coding was complete, codes were reorganized, which involved combining duplicate codes and organizing codes into thematic hierarchies that allowed for easier visualization and contextualization of the data (Bernard, 2011).

9.5 OVERVIEW OF RESULTS AND DISCUSSION

Quantitative assessment of nutrient adequacy indicated that 55% (n = 33) of the participants in the sample were found to have inadequate intakes of calcium and 61% (n = 37) were found to have inadequate intakes of vitamin D when compared to the EAR for age. When perceptions of intake were integrated with the FFQ data, more than half of the young adults in this study perceived themselves as adequate consumers of calcium (57%, n = 19/33) and vitamin D (78%, n = 29/37), when they were inadequate according to the FFQ.

When the qualitative data were considered, two themes can be identified that helped contextualize participants' beliefs in the adequacy of their intakes: nutrition misinformation and nutrition as a low priority. Participants showed poor knowledge of the sources of vitamin D and calcium. Participants located calcium and vitamin D in more foods than they actually are present in, which led them to perceive their intake as greater than it actually was. "[I get enough] because it's in everything I eat. It's in the cheese that I have on everything. It's in milk that I drink straight. It's in vegetables when I eat them" (Male, 29, Graduate). The view of these nutrients as ubiquitous led participants to assume that general food consumption, especially of healthy foods, would provide enough nutrients. "Yup. I think [I get enough]. Because I eat my greens and I eat my veggies and I get enough sun" (Male, 26, College). Additionally, the labeling of calcium and vitamin D as micronutrients led participants to think that they only needed to be present in their diets in small amounts and so it was easy to obtain enough without actively seeking out these nutrients.

The second theme is more general and concerns the low priority that most participants placed on nutrition. These young adults were generally not concerned about nutritional content of foods as a factor that affected their food purchasing. In fact, nutrition was placed as a low priority unless it was tangentially related to another interest, such as fitness or weight loss. "I don't think at the moment it's directly important just because I'm young and I don't really think about that kind of stuff" (Female, 24, University). Perhaps their age and lack of previous medical problems made health a low priority for them. Nutrition was viewed as nonessential for their current life stage as it could be corrected when they were older and it became more important to eat healthfully. As one participant indicated, nutrition was only considered when it was connected to weight loss. "The first thing I look at is the fat and calories. I don't pay attention to any sort of the percentage of other nutrients that they have" (Male, 28, College). This statement echoes the sentiment of many participants who saw nutrition as an intervention for weight loss or fitness, rather than a daily priority.

Overall, the qualitative results suggest that the participants' perceptions of dietary adequacy can be linked to their overall knowledge about nutrition and their beliefs about specific nutrients. Since they perceive their intake of calcium and vitamin D to be higher than it actually is, this is an issue to address in future communications. Raising awareness means reaching those young adults who believe their intake is adequate and encouraging them to question their consumption practices and to listen to prevention education. At the same time, the results suggest that current prevention education targeting older adults and individuals who are already concerned about their intake will not be effective with these younger adults as they do not perceive themselves as being at risk of inadequate calcium and vitamin D intake.

Information needs to be connected to topics that interest young adults, such as fitness or weight loss, in order to catch and hold their attention to nutrition as a whole. Targeting Canadian young adults means designing education that promotes awareness of calcium and vitamin D consumption in individuals who do not consider themselves at risk and encouraging individuals to question their intake before presenting them with nutrition information.

9.6 CHALLENGES AND LIMITATIONS

An issue that was at the forefront of the challenges experienced in this study was the difficulty in determining how to integrate the results in order to speak to the research question as a whole (Burke Johnson and Onwuegbuzie, 2004; Caracelli and Greene, 1993; Creswell, 2008; Onwuegbuzie and Leech, 2006; Teddlie and Tashakkori, 2003). Since each method measured something that was fundamentally different, bringing them together posed a problem. The methods were not simply two ways of measuring the same phenomenon and the data types themselves contained very different limitations. Identifying how these methods could be used in tandem required recognizing that they provided different perspectives on the research question and together could be used to explain the problem. The research question sought to explore how young adults understood their perceived intake in comparison to their actual intake, with a focus on why there might be discrepancies. The FFQs gave a sense of how much calcium and vitamin D young adults were consuming, which provided a measurement of their actual intake. The interview data provided the information on their perceptions, using a series of questions that ranged from the explicit to more general questions surrounding the importance of calcium and vitamin D to help provide context for their actual intake. The degree to which young adults understood their nutrition and considered micronutrients as an aspect of nutrition could provide the context for how reliable their assessment of their own intake was and, when specifically explored in the young adults that over- or underconsumed calcium and vitamin D, could aid in explaining the observed patterns.

While the outcome of this study revealed the importance of using a mixed methods approach, there were a number of inherent challenges. In order to maximize data collection, the FFQs and interviews were conducted at the same time, so that the FFQs were monitored and no data points were lost. In this case participants had to complete all three parts of the study or the data could not be used, which made it time-intensive. The interviews were concerned with broad beliefs and the FFQs were designed only to measure reported intake. Integrating the two required careful design of a research question that incorporated the types of data generated by each method.

The methods themselves contain inherent limitations. The FFQ required participants to recall their intake over the past month and then reduced it down to a single measurement of daily intake. This has the potential to misrepresent participants' actual intake of calcium and vitamin D. Interviews are also subject to a series of commonly experienced limitations as described by Bernard (2011). Calculating vitamin D is problematic as vitamin D is both consumed and synthesized after exposure to UVB radiation, however, this limitation was mediated by administering the FFQs only during the winter months when vitamin D cannot be synthesized.

The importance of the research question to a mixed methods approach is underscored by Onwuegbuzie and Leech (2006), since the design of the research question dictates the methods and analysis. When the intention from the outset is to blend methods, the research question had to be formulated to take advantage of the specific types of data that the methods can generate. A broad, exploratory research question that contained a comparative question was found to be more conducive to data amalgamation than a specific question as it created more space for probing relationships and allowing for questions concerning the "how" and "why" of food consumption patterns (Onwuegbuzie and Leech, 2006).

The decision to use the qualitative data to create context for the quantitative data follows accepted procedures for mixed methods, where data is integrated in phases that begin with one data type informing the collection of the second data type (Driscoll et al., 2007; Onwuegbuzie and Leech, 2006). In this case the quantitative data was collected first, which allowed for the qualitative data to build upon the initial results through inductive exploration of the topic. This approach minimized the risk of one method overwhelming the other and did not preference one approach or data set over the other; each was treated as equally valuable and revealing.

One of the major concerns was the potential that contradictory data would pose for analysis. This issue was mediated by the use of broad, open-ended questions in the interviews in order to generate data that could be used to explore multiple different FFQ results. However, contradictory data is not necessarily a problem as it could indicate that the issue being investigated is more complex than the research question or analysis allows for. While this approach could be viewed as limiting the detail that could be gathered, it allowed for integration of the data in a meaningful way that could later be used to create more detailed questions once larger trends had been established. Ongoing assessment of the FFQs during the data collection process and immediate transcription and cursory analysis of the interviews were essential in ensuring the two data sets could be used together.

9.7 EPISTEMOLOGICAL QUESTIONS IN MIXED METHODS: VALIDITY AND RELIABILITY

The concepts of validity and reliability frame the understanding of contemporary scientific research and, for this reason, warrant a specific discussion here. The issues of validity and reliability underscore all qualitative and quantitative studies, but represent standards that are much more difficult for qualitative studies to meet. Validity is a measurement of the accuracy of data, which is the degree to which a technique measures what it is designed to measure (Burrows et al., 2010; Quandt, 1986). From the positivist perspective, validity is the degree to which a method provides the objective truth which, from a scientific standpoint, is understood to both exist and be attainable through the correct methodologies (Golafshani, 2003). Reliability is the ability to obtain the same result every time the method is repeated (Quandt, 1986). While both FFQs and interviews rely on self-reported data, which has known limitations, the FFQ can be subjected to the standard tests of validity and replicability as it is possible to know the amount of calcium/vitamin D consumed and to repeat this measurement successfully as the amount of calcium/vitamin D should not change significantly provided all variables remain consistent. Since FFQs are limited by the potential for retrospective errors and the self-reported nature of the method, they often require validation using additional methods (Burrows et al., 2010; Johnson, 2010; Krall et al., 1988). Previous tests of validation on the FFQ used here have supported its use in a young adult Canadian population, as the FFQ was combined with 7-day food diaries and repeated with large sample sizes on multiple occasions (Wu et al., 2009).

Problems emerge when the standards of validity and reliability are applied to qualitative methods as they are interested in the attitudes, beliefs, perceptions, and experiences of individuals and so it becomes more difficult to satisfy validity and reliability (Hart et al., 2002; Ulijaszek, 2004). The assumption of an objective truth that underlies validity is more difficult to apply to personal opinions regarding abstract concepts. There is often no knowable objective truth and looking for an objective truth lies outside the assumptions on which most qualitative methods are based. Qualitative methods, such as interviews and focus groups, are concerned with the process of how people create meaning through their experiences and perceptions of the world (Golafshani, 2003; Hubert, 2004; Pope and Mays, 1995; Sofaer, 1999). The goal is to describe these processes and to identify the common themes that underlie them. Using a standard that requires an objective truth misconstrues the purpose of using a qualitative method (Golafshani, 2003). A similar problem exists for reliability because people are not static. People live in a state of "being in" the world and as a result their perceptions are constantly being affected by their experiences (Bernard, 2011). Qualitative data are not designed to be subjected to the same standards of replicability, since individual beliefs and perceptions can change, even as a consequence of discussing them with an interviewer. While this type of data provides essential context to intangible phenomena, its results are less generalizable than those achieved using quantitative data. So while the FFQ data may be replicated in other populations, the interview and pile sort data may differ because populations are different or because perceptions change making its applicability more limited.

Using a mixed methods approach therefore involves rethinking the positivist principles that underlie approaches to research design and accepting that the contributions that qualitative research can make are a direct result of the type of data produced. Rather than holding all methods to the same scientific standards of validity and replicability it is important to recognize the limitations of both data types and use them in ways that most effectively draw on their strengths. Interviews and pile sorts should not be used to identify objective truths in perceptions, but to provide essential context for understanding the intake behaviors identified in the FFQs. While these results are not necessarily generalizable and may change with individual experiences, this does not detract from the ability of interviews to explain the context of the specific reported intake values and to aid in drawing conclusions about behaviors.

9.8 CONCLUSION

The importance of collecting data using multiple methods is paramount as multiple lines of evidence both strengthen results and introduce new perspectives. The challenges inherent in a mixed methods approach need to be recognized and considered because mediating them must be integrated into the design of a study, not just in analysis and interpretation. Uniting disparate lines of data requires the researcher to think carefully about the research question, theory, methodology, and analysis in order to be familiar with the specific strengths and limitations of the methods and frameworks that are being applied. The pragmatic theory that underlies mixed methods recognizes the need to compromise between data types in order to create a whole that draws on the preferred traits from each method and combines them in a way that generates new and interesting perspectives on the research question. When applied to anthropological questions, and specifically to food studies, the desired outcome is a melding of the social and biological that speaks to actual practices and social beliefs.

The application of a mixed methods approach to this case study allowed a more nuanced understanding of how young adults develop and apply beliefs about nutrition to their consumption processes. Integral to the exploration of this issue was the ability to apply two different types of data to a single research question in order to create multifaceted results. What emerged from this process was information on both the nutritional adequacy of the young adult respondents and the perceptions and beliefs that underlie nutrient consumption and directly influence adequacy. The same population was used to collect both sets of data in this study, rather than conducting separate studies on different populations, and so inferences can be made about correlation. The identification of this context means that more detailed recommendations, beyond simply increasing education, can be made for the creation of programs that directly address nutrient inadequacy of comparable Canadian young adults. The contribution of mixed methods in this context was the generation of a dataset that provided social context for food intake on a single study population in order to show how perceptions can influence action and create tangible recommendations for change.

While there are limitations to using mixed methods and it is not suitable for all data types or research questions, the benefits of such an approach are invaluable in accessing the complexity of human behavior. Quantitative studies can produce measurable information on human behaviors, but applying this information or modifying behaviors requires going beyond observation to access meaning in order to identify ways of instigating change. The use of mixed methods offers the tools for a more efficient and dynamic study of human behavior.

ACKNOWLEDGMENTS

This project would not have been possible without the support of my supervisor Dr. Tina Moffat and my committee members Dr. Stephanie Atkinson and Dr. Megan Brickley. Thank you to Gretel Pelto and the other reviewers who have contributed their invaluable comments to this paper. Lastly, thank you to my coeditor Madeleine Mant for her support through all phases of this project.

REFERENCES

Atkinson, S.A., 2011. Defining the process of dietary reference intakes: framework for the United States and Canada. Am. J. Clin. Nutr. 94, 655S–667S.

Becker, W., Welten, D., 2001. Under-reporting in dietary surveys—implications for development of food-based dietary guidelines. Public Health Nutr. 4, 683–687.

Bernard, H., 2011. Research Methods in Anthropology. AltaMira, Maryland.

Briefel, R.R., Sempos, C.T., McDowell, M.A., Chien, S., Alaimo, K., 1997. Dietary methods research in the third National Health and Nutrition Examination Survey: underreporting of energy intake. Am. J. Clin. Nutr. 65, 1203S–1209S.

Burke Johnson, R., Onwuegbuzie, A., 2004. Mixed methods research: a research paradigm whose time has come. Educ. Res. 33, 14–26.

Burrows, T.L., Martin, R.J., Collins, C.E., 2010. A systematic review of the validity of dietary assessment methods in children when compared with the method of doubly labeled water. J. Am. Diet. Assoc. 110, 1501–1510.

Caracelli, V.J., Greene, J.C., 1993. Data analysis strategies for mixed method evaluation designs. Educ. Eval. Policy Anal. 15, 195–207.

Cook, A., Pryer, J., Shetty, P., 2000. The problem of accuracy in dietary surveys. Analysis of the over 65 UK national diet and nutrition survey. J. Epidemiol. Community Health 54, 611–616.

Creed-Kanashiro, H.M., Bartolini, R.M., Fukumoto, M.N., Uribe, T.G., Robert, R.C., Bentley, M.E., 2003. Formative research to develop a nutrition education intervention to improve dietary iron intake among women and adolescent girls through community kitchens in Lima, Peru. J. Nutr. 133, 3987S–3991S.

Creswell, J.W., 2008. Research Design: Qualitative, Quantitative, and Mixed Methods Approaches. Sage, London.

de Garine, I., 2004. Anthropology of food and pluridisciplinarity. In: Macbeth, H., MacClancy, J. (Eds.), Researching Food Habits. Berghahn Books, New York, pp. 15–28.

Driscoll, D.L., Appiah-Yeboah, A., Salib, P., Rupert, D.J., 2007. Merging qualitative and quantitative data in mixed methods research: how to and why not. Ecol. Environ. Anthropol. 3, 19–28.

Edstrom, K.M., Devine, C.M., 2001. Consistency in women's orientations to food and nutrition in midlife and older age: a 10-year qualitative follow-up. J. Nutr. Educ. 33, 215–223.

Garriguet, D., 2008. Under-reporting of Energy Intake in the Canadian Community Heath Survey. Statistics, Canada, Ottawa.

Golafshani, N., 2003. Understanding reliability and validity in qualitative research. Qual. Rep. 8, 597–607.

Hart, K.H., Bishop, J.A., Truby, H., 2002. An investigation into school children's knowledge and awareness of food and nutrition. J. Hum. Nutr. Diet. 15, 129–140.

Health Canada, 2012. Do Canadian Adults Meet Their Nutrient Requirements Through Food Intake Alone? Health Canada, Ottawa.

Hubert, A., 2004. Qualitative research in the anthropology of food: a comprehensive qualitative/quantitative approach. In: Macbeth, H., MacClancy, J. (Eds.), Researching Food Habits. Berghahn Books, New York.

IOM, 2000. Dietary Reference Intakes: Applications to Dietary Assessment. Institute of Medicine, Washington, DC.

IOM, 2010. Dietary Reference Intakes for Calcium and Vitamin D. The National Academies Press.

Johnson, R., 2010. Dietary intake: how do we measure what people are really eating? Obes. Res. 10, 63S–68S.

Johnson, R., Onwuegbuzie, J., Turner, L.A., 2007. Toward a definition of mixed methods research. J. Mix. Methods Res. 1, 112–133.

Johnston, F., 1987. Nutritional Anthropology. Alan Liss, New York.

Krall, E.A., Dwyer, J.T., Coleman, K.A., 1988. Factors influencing accuracy of dietary recall. Nutr. Res. 8, 829–841.

Macbeth, H., MacClancy, J., 2004. Researching Food Habits. Berghahn Books, New York.

MacClancy, J., Macbeth, H., 2004. How to do anthropologies of food. In: Macbeth, H., MacClancy, J. (Eds.), Researching Food Habits. Berghahn Books, New York, pp. 1–14.

McGarvey, S., 2009. Interdisciplinary translational research in anthropology, nutrition and public health. Annu. Rev. Anthropol. 38, 233–249.

McPherson, R.S., Hoelscher, D., Alexander, M., Scanlon, K.S., Serdula, M., 2000. Dietary assessment methods among school-aged children: validity and reliability. Prev. Med. 31, S11–S33.

Onwuegbuzie, A., Leech, N.L., 2006. Linking research questions to mixed methods data analysis procedures. Qual. Rep. 11, 474–498.

Pelto, G.H., Goodman, A.H., Dufour, D.L., 2000. The biocultural perspective in nutritional anthropology. In: Goodman, A.H., Dufour, D.L., Pelto, G.H. (Eds.), Nutritional Anthropology: Biocultural Perspectives on Food and Nutrition. Mayfield, California, pp. 1–9.

Pope, C., Mays, N., 1995. Reaching the parts other methods cannot reach: an introduction to qualitative methods in health and health services research. BMJ 311, 42–45.

Quandt, S.A., 1986. Nutritional anthropology: the individual focus. In: Quandt, S.A., Rittenbaugh, C. (Eds.), Training Manual in Nutritional Anthropology. American Anthropological Association, Washington D.C., pp. 3−20.

Quintiliani, L.M., Campbell, M.K., Haines, P.S., Webber, K.H., 2008. The use of the pile sort method in identifying groups of healthful lifestyle behaviours among female community college students. J. Am. Diet. Assoc. 108, 1503−1507.

Rizek, R.L., Pao, E.M., 1990. Dietary intake methodology I. USDA surveys and supporting research. J. Nutr. 120, 1525−1529.

Sofaer, S., 1999. Qualitative methods: what are they and why use them? Health Serv. Res. 34, 1101−1118.

Teddlie, C., Tashakkori, A., 2003. Major issues and controversies in the use of mixed methods in the social and behavioural sciences. In: Tashakkori, A., Teddlie, C. (Eds.), Handbook of Mixed Methods in Social and Behavioural Research. Sage, California, pp. 3−50.

Ulijaszek, S.J., 2004. Dietary intake methods in the anthropology of food and nutrition. In: Macbeth, H., MacClancy, J. (Eds.), Researching Food Habits. Berghahn Books, New York, pp. 119−134.

Vallianatos, H., Raine, K., 2008. Consuming food and constructing identities among Arabic and South Asian immigrant women. Food Cult. Soc. 2, 356−373.

Whiting, S.J., Langlois, K.A., Vatanparast, H., Greene-Finestone, L.S., 2011. The vitamin D status of Canadians relative to the 2011 Dietary Reference Intakes: an examination in children and adults with and without supplement use. Am. J. Clin. Nutr. 94, 128−135. Available from: http://dx.doi.org/10.3945/ajcn.111.013268.

Wilson, C.S., 2002. Reasons for eating: personal experiences in nutrition and anthropology. Appetite 38, 63−67.

Wu, H., Gozdzik, A., Barta, J.L., Wagner, D., Cole, D.E., Vieth, R., et al., 2009. The development and evaluation of a food frequency questionnaire used in assessing vitamin D intake in a sample of health young Canadian adults of diverse ancestry. Nutr. Res. 29, 255−261.

CHAPTER 10

Conclusions and Future Directions: Converging Disparate Approaches in a New Biological Anthropology

C. de la Cova[1,2]
[1]Department of Anthropology, University of South Carolina, Columbia, SC, United States
[2]African American Studies Program, University of South Carolina, Columbia, SC, United States

Scholars of biological anthropology, and its subdiscipline of bioarchaeology, are uniquely situated to provide innovative knowledge on the relationship between biology, health, environment, identity, and the social conditions of past and current populations. However, for this scholarship to be convincing, effective, and applicable, researchers must move beyond one-dimensional analyses that solely discuss metrics, anomalies, pathologies, DNA presence, and nutrient intake. Bioarchaeologist Jane Buikstra (1977) was one of the first scholars to advocate skeletal analyses be situated within a cross-disciplinary and multimethodological framework that included cultural and environmental variables. Three years later Buikstra and colleague Della Cook (1980) stressed the utilization of a biocultural approach that addressed how social status and culture affected mortuary practices and skeletal disease processes. Cook (1981) later emphasized the importance of recognizing regional and historic factors in regard to biological differences associated with social status. Better methodological frameworks have emerged in recent years to assist biological anthropologists in environmentally, culturally, and socially contextualizing their research (Goodman and Leatherman, 1998; Goodman et al., 1988; Goodman and Martin, 2002; Klaus, 2012; Martin et al., 2013; Zuckerman and Armelagos, 2011).

However, cross-disciplinary analyses still remain underutilized by bioanthropologists. Emphasis is often placed on methodologies that address biological differences and pathologies. Thus, the individual(s) studied becomes silenced and subsequently the embodiment of

Beyond the Bones. DOI: http://dx.doi.org/10.1016/B978-0-12-804601-2.00010-7

their disorders, diseases, and differences. This results in a disconnect between the biological remains, social context, and identity of the deceased (Sofaer, 2006). Scholars of the new bioarchaeology, however, have advocated for improved integration of biological, social, behavioral, and ecological research (Agarwal and Glencross, 2011). Sabrina Agarwal and Bonnie Glencross (2011, p. 3) indicate that the "goal of this new bioarchaeological practice is to transcend the skeletal body into the realm of lived experience and to make a significant contribution to our understanding of social processes and life in the past."

The best way to resocialize and rehumanize archaeological groups is through the incorporation of disparate lines of data and diverse methodologies that force the researcher to think beyond the bones to factors that comprise the lived experience of the individual(s) under analyses. This groundbreaking book, *Beyond the Bones*, illustrates, through thorough descriptions of cross-disciplinary approaches and disparate data sets, how this can be done so future researchers can conduct holistic and multidimensional skeletal biology-related analyses. Each chapter utilizes multiple methodologies and a diversity of data sets, including demographic sources, cemetery records, DNA, clinical research, historical documents, censuses, hospital records, public health data, linguistic models, migration information, and nutritional data. Whether it be comprehending the coevolution of Tanoan-speaking Pueblo Indians through the analysis of linguistic, genetic, and craniometrics relationships as discussed by Schillaci and Wichmann (see chapter: The Use of Linguistic Data in Bioarchaeological Research: An Example From the American Southwest), or reconciling historical documents, epidemiological data, environmental sources, and skeletal findings, like many scholars in this volume, including Murphy (see chapter: Fifty Shades of Grey Literature: Deconstructing "High" Infant Mortality With New Data Sets in Historic Cemetery Populations), Mant (see chapter: "Readmitted Under Urgent Circumstance": Uniting Archives and Bioarchaeology at the Royal London Hospital), Reusch (see chapter: Reading Between the Lines: Disparate Data and Castration Studies), and Marciniak (see chapter: Hunting for Pathogens: Ancient DNA and the Historical Record), each author demonstrates how these disparate lines of evidence can be woven together to create a holistic interpretation of paleopathological and skeletal findings.

Murphy, Mant, Reusch, and Marciniak illustrate the importance of consulting primary historical sources when examining groups with a documented past. These authors demonstrate the detailed information these data can provide in demographic, paleopathological, and DNA analysis. Murphy (see chapter: Fifty Shades of Grey Literature: Deconstructing "High" Infant Mortality With New Data Sets in Historic Cemetery Populations) discovers that, contrary to the high infant mortality rates archaeologists associated with past groups, historic cemetery data provides plausible low to moderate infant mortality rates comparable to those reported by historical demographers. Mant (see chapter: "Readmitted Under Urgent Circumstance": Uniting Archives and Bioarchaeology at the Royal London Hospital) discusses the importance of primary sources and the limitations of paleopathological samples in her Royal London Hospital analysis. Health-related documents provide a wealth of information, including diagnosis, cause of illness or trauma, occupation, possible residence, and social status of the individual(s) studied. Inferring social position allows the researcher to push beyond medical records, to reconstruct possible lifeways, access to resources, and what limiting factors may have impacted the health. If archaeological evidence, public health records, or other historical resources are present, these data can also be incorporated.

Reusch (see chapter: Reading Between the Lines: Disparate Data and Castration Studies) integrates historical data with numerous disparate sources to address castration, which is rarely discussed in the skeletal biological literature. Pulling from archaeological, zooarchaeological, paleopathological, anthropological, ethnological, medical, historical, and musical data, Reusch creates a temporally and biologically multifaceted methodology to locate and identify castrates in the bioarchaeological record. This approach narrows the historic time periods and geographic locations associated with eunuchs and elaborates on the skeletal changes observed in prepubertally castrated skeletons, including elongated long bones, kyphosis, and other modifications in the pelvis and skull. Reusch's research also forces skeletal biologists to consider the interaction between culture, gender identity, and status.

This volume also demonstrates how the disparate data can be utilized to address limitations inherent in bioanthropological data with a historical context (Mant and Marciniak). All skeletal collections, including archaeological remains, have undergone different selective or preservational processes that make them unrepresentative of a normal population. These factors need to be addressed by the researcher. As Mant discovered, fracture rates in her skeletal samples were less severe and less varied than those documented in hospital records, which were more severe and affected mobility. She also observed more leg-related trauma in hospital documents and higher rates of broken ribs in her skeletal sample. Documentary evidence indicated that rib fractures were not considered serious enough to warrant hospital entry. Furthermore, dissection-related activities at the Royal London Hospital may have affected the composition of the skeletal sample.

Whilst Mant's findings highlight how collections can be biased (or underrepresentative) and disparate data sources can provide a more holistic picture of past groups, they also stress how these sources need to be evaluated. Recorded information associated with documented collections should be viewed with caution. Age-data is especially problematic as most past groups did not keep birth records. Occupation data may also be inaccurate. Furthermore, the researcher must always be conscious of the role social status plays in the creation of documented skeletal collections (de la Cova, 2012, 2014; Muller et al., 2016).

Marciniak (see chapter: Hunting for Pathogens: Ancient DNA and the Historical Record) also illustrates how historical records, especially those associated with the Roman Empire, need to be evaluated carefully to determine what constitutes known present-day illnesses. Her study, like Reusch's, relies on a plethora of disparate sources to argue that DNA molecular data, like osteological research, must be examined within the historical, archaeological, literary, cultural, and environmental contexts of the individuals being sequenced. These factors explain environmental-related illnesses, disease treatment, hygienic processes, and the impact landscape has on disease risk and exposure.

Other scholars in this volume stress the importance of integrating clinical and paleopathological research (Lockau, see chapter: The Present Informs the Past: Incorporating Modern Clinical Data Into Paleopathological Analyses of Metabolic Bone Disease). Skeletal biologists can only observe diseases and disorders after they have affected the skeleton, whereas clinicians see all the subtle nuances of illnesses and deficiencies, how they vary and progress through multiple stages in the soft tissue and skeleton, and their environmental and genetic causative factors. Biological anthropologists should, as Lockau emphasizes, actively engage with this literature to better comprehend how disorders present in both the soft tissue and the skeleton. Scholars should also consult clinical literature to better comprehend environmental causations of illness.

Disparate sources are not only the result of cross-disciplinary research. Jelena Bekvalac (see chapter: Direct Digital Radiographic Imaging of Archaeological Skeletal Assemblages: An Advantageous Technique and the Use of the Images as a Research Resource) describes digital disparate data sets that are key to osteological investigation. These include osteological databases, digital imaging, direct digital radiography, computed tomography scanning, and 3D modeling. These methods allow bioarchaeologists to see beyond the bones, to their surface textures, shapes, and internal structures. All are imperative for advanced paleopathological diagnosis and nondestructive analyses of skeletal material. Scholars can also digitally scan remains for future study, thus minimalizing handling and damage.

Utilizing these disparate data sets allows the bioanthropologist to see beyond the skeleton to the lived experience. However, as a discipline, we should strive to not only understand the past, but connect our research to the present. Holland's (see chapter: Uniting Perception and Reality in Human Nutrition: Integration of Qualitative and Quantitative Data to Understand Consumption) examination of the social and cultural perceptions of vitamin D intake is applicable to both the past and present, as it is likely past groups, like contemporary students, did not comprehend the nutritional importance of vitamin D or the role it plays in bone maintenance.

Beyond the Bones clearly illustrates that disease, trauma, biological stress, and other anomalies and pathologies do not affect the skeleton in a vacuum. It emphasizes the importance of examining disparate lines of data in order to synthesize the complex interactions between skeletal biology, pathology, disease, nutrition, culture, and environment. Furthermore, the authors detail their methods and clearly explain the disparate sources utilized and their limitations. When read as a whole, *Beyond the Bones* provides various approaches on how to utilize multidimensional, cross-disciplinary research designs that integrate diverse disparate data sets. Each study reanimates and rehumanizes the individuals examined, placing them within their environmental, social, and cultural contexts and illustrating how these factors impacted their skeletal health. It is imperative that biological anthropologists embrace these methodological approaches, which are central to the new bioarchaeology. Questions related to the impact of physical environs, culture, status, societal perception, or marginalization and stigmatization by society must be addressed using disparate sources so a more holistic social bioarchaeology can emerge.

REFERENCES

Agarwal, S.C., Glencross, B.A. (Eds.), 2011. Social Bioarchaeology. Wiley-Blackwell, Malden, MA.

Buikstra, J.E., 1977. Differential diagnosis: an epidemiological model. Yearb. Phys. Anthropol. 20, 316–328.

Buikstra, J.E., Cook, D.C., 1980. Palaeopathology: an American account. Annu. Rev. Anthropol. 9, 433–470.

Cook, D.C., 1981. Mortality, age structure, and status in the interpretation of stress indicators in prehistoric skeletons: a dental example from the Lower Illinois Valley. In: Chapman, R., Kinnes, I., Randsborg, K. (Eds.), The Archaeology of Death. Cambridge University Press, Cambridge, pp. 133–144.

de la Cova, C., 2012. Trauma patterns in 19th-century-born African American and Euro-American females. Int. J. Paleopathol. 2, 61–68.

de la Cova, C., 2014. The biological effects of urbanization and in-migration on 19th-century-born African Americans and Euro-Americans of low socioeconomic status: an anthropological and historical approach. In: Zuckerman, M.K. (Ed.), Are Modern Environments Bad for Human Health? Revisiting the Second Epidemiological Transition. Wiley-Blackwell, Malden, MA, pp. 243–266.

Goodman, A.H., Thomas, R.B., Swedlund, A.C., Armelagos, G.J., 1988. Biocultural perspectives on stress in prehistoric, historical and contemporary population research. Yearb. Phys. Anthropol. 31, 169–202.

Goodman, A.H., Leatherman, T.L., 1998. Building a New Biocultural Synthesis: Political-Economic Perspectives on Human Biology. The University of Michigan Press, Ann Arbor, MI.

Goodman, A., Martin, D., 2002. Reconstructing health profiles from skeletal remains. In: Steckel, R., Rose, J. (Eds.), The Backbone of History: Health and Nutrition in the Western Hemisphere. Cambridge University Press, Cambridge, pp. 11–61.

Klaus, H.D., 2012. The bioarchaeology of structural violence: a theoretical model and a case study. In: Martin, D.L., Harrod, R.P. (Eds.), The Bioarchaeology of Violence. University Press of Florida, Gainesville, FL, pp. 29–62.

Martin, D.L., Harrod, R.P., Pérez, V.R., 2013. Bioarchaeology: An Integrated Approach to Working With Human Remains. Springer Press, New York, NY.

Muller, J.L., Pearlstein, K.E., de la Cova, C., 2016. Dissection and documented skeletal collections. In: Nystrom, K. (Ed.), The Bioarchaeology of Dissection and Autopsy in the United States. Springer, New York, NY, pp. 185–201.

Sofaer, J.R., 2006. The Body as Material Culture: A Theoretical Osteoarchaeology. Cambridge University Press, Cambridge.

Zuckerman, M.K., Armelagos, G.J., 2011. The origins of biocultural dimensions in bioarchaeology. In: Agarwal, S.C., Glencross, B.A. (Eds.), Social Bioarchaeology. Wiley-Blackwell, Malden, MA, pp. 15–43.

Printed in the United States
By Bookmasters